Sites of Violence, Sites of Grace

Sites of Violence, Sites of Grace

Christian Nonviolence and the Traumatized Self

Cynthia Hess

LEXINGTON BOOKS

A division of
ROWMAN & LITTLEFIELD PUBLISHERS, INC.
Lanham • Boulder • New York • Toronto • Plymouth, UK

LEXINGTON BOOKS

A division of Rowman & Littlefield Publishers, Inc.
A wholly owned subsidiary of The Rowman & Littlefield Publishing Group, Inc.
4501 Forbes Boulevard, Suite 200
Lanham, MD 20706

Estover Road
Plymouth PL6 7PY
United Kingdom

British Library Cataloguing in Publication Information Available

Library of Congress Cataloging-in-Publication Data

Hess, Cynthia, 1971-
Sites of violence, sites of grace : Christian nonviolence and the traumatized self / Cynthia Hess.
p. cm.
Includes bibliographical references and index.
ISBN-13: 978-0-7391-1945-7 (cloth : alk. paper)
ISBN-10: 0-7391-1945-1 (cloth : alk. paper)
ISBN-13: 978-0-7391-3083-4 (electronic)
ISBN-10: 0-7391-3083-8 (electronic)
1. Nonviolence—Religious aspects—Christianity. 2. Psychic trauma—Religious aspects—Christianity. 3. Church. 4. Yoder, John Howard. I. Title.

BT736.6.H47 2009
241'.697--dc2 2008034400

Printed in the United States of America

∞™ The paper used in this publication meets the minimum requirements of American National Standard for Information Sciences—Permanence of Paper for Printed Library Materials, ANSI/NISO Z39.48–1992.

Contents

Acknowledgments

Many people have given me the kind of support and guidance that make it possible to complete a project of this nature. Shannon Craigo-Snell and Serene Jones advised the dissertation that formed the basis for this book, offering invaluable input along the way. Marilyn Adams generously read early drafts of the chapters and gave helpful comments that sharpened and clarified their arguments. My colleagues at Yale provided companionship and challenging theological conversation; I am particularly indebted to Jennifer Beste and Jill Carlson Colwell for their insights about trauma and theology. Claudia Muro's good humor and kind spirit helped to make our home a peaceful retreat. The late Anne Zirkle embodied a passion for theological reflection that was an inspiration to me, first during our time at Davidson College and then at Yale. Without her friendship I would not have written this book. And the late Jill Hungerford enlivened my early years in New Haven with her sheer energy, joy of life, and good-natured appreciation for my "Pennsylvania Dutch-isms."

Others contributed to this project in invaluable but different ways. I especially thank the four trauma survivors who agreed to be interviewed about their experiences of healing; their honesty, wisdom, and courage helped me to see more clearly the possibility of hope and the strength of the human spirit. Karl Plank offered classes at Davidson that cultivated my interest in trauma and theology, and I am grateful for his continuing guidance and friendship. Zama Coursen-Neff has also provided life-giving friendship over the years; our occasional weekend visits in New York and New Haven were welcome breaks that renewed my energy to write. St. Mary's College of Maryland gave me the opportunity to teach some of the material in this book, and Virginia Theological Seminary graciously allowed me to use their library for much of the research. Maera Winters at Lexingon Books also provided valuable editorial assistance along the way, and Kaudie McLean prepared the index with diligence and care.

I am grateful as well to my family for their support over the years. Jim Hess, Sue Hess, Steve Hess, and Nancy Hess have created a loving family network that is an amazing gift. The Edmondsons and Reids have extended this network in recent years. Finally, I am most indebted to my spouse, Stephen Edmondson. In addition to being a wonderful parent to our sons, Andrew and Christopher, he has patiently read and re-read more drafts of this book than I am sure either of us can remember. At times when I felt overwhelmed by the daunting nature of this peculiar undertaking, he offered wise counsel and keen theological insights that shaped the final product in crucial ways. Without his support, I doubt that I would have arrived at this point where I can finally replace my oft-repeated refrain of "someday it will be done" with "it *is* done."

Introduction

Over the past several years, the so-called war on terror has caused the question of nonviolence to loom large in the minds of many North American scholars and activists. A spirited debate has arisen about whether nonviolence can offer an effective way of responding to the violence of the contemporary era.[1] Some individuals find it hard to imagine that nonviolence has a place in our world today—a world in which people fly planes into buildings and explode their own cars, all for the sake of taking human life. Others, however, believe that it is precisely in such a world that nonviolence must persist. The very existence of this debate indicates that nonviolence is not simply a "thing of the past," something to be studied in history books that describe the lives of great individuals like Mohandas Gandhi and Martin Luther King, Jr. Instead, nonviolence is alive and well—for some, as an ethic that must be recalled in order to be dismissed, and for others, as a way of life that even today holds a very real possibility for transformation.

My own commitments fall on the side of those who endorse the latter position. This is due, partly, I suspect, to my upbringing in the Church of the Brethren, one of the historic Christian "peace churches." Although my reflections on nonviolence certainly include moments of doubt about its potential effectiveness and whether it is always "right," I share the conviction of the peace churches that nonviolence remains essential to the Christian life and to the task of transforming violence and the terror it generates. At the same time, the challenges of the contemporary era have pushed me to think more deeply about the meaning of nonviolence and the multiple ways it is practiced. Over the years I have found that the Christian traditions contain rich resources for such reflection: The early Christians, the eleventh-century "Peace of God" movement in France, the Waldenses, Lollards, and

Moravian Brethren of the later Middle Ages, and the sixteenth-century Anabaptists and seventeenth-century Quakers represent just some of the groups that have given nonviolence a vital, if minority, place within Christianity. In the twentieth-century people as diverse as Martin Luther King, Jr., Walter Wink, Dorothee Solle, the Catholic Workers, and Desmond Tutu have kept this tradition alive by endorsing nonviolence as a way of life that can promote authentic social transformation.

Within the contemporary era, John Howard Yoder has presented an argument for nonviolence that has been particularly influential for both the historic peace churches and for some mainstream Christians. In Yoder's understanding, the biblical narratives show that the moral character of God is revealed in Jesus' nonviolence and refusal to dominate his enemies with sheer force. Since Jesus reveals God's character, Christians must follow after him. The kind of community Jesus formed is, therefore, what the church is called to be. The church must live as a community that enacts relationships that differ from the ones found in the wider society—relationships in which social hierarchies are relativized, enemies are reconciled, and persons of diverse backgrounds can live together in peace.

While Yoder offers a powerful vision of nonviolence, it is my contention that his work overlooks a dimension of violence that contemporary understandings of nonviolence must address. Yoder's writings on nonviolence focus primarily on pacifism and the refusal of military violence, which, as J. Denny Weaver observes, historically have been central concerns of the Mennonite tradition out of which Yoder operates.[2] In focusing on these concerns, Yoder's work clarifies how nonviolence can respond to what some scholars call "external" violence, forms of violent harm that assault people from without. But it does not bring into view what others describe as "internal" or "internalized" violence, forms of violence that have assaulted persons from the outside and then moved into their bodies, minds, and souls. According to bell hooks, Lisa Adler, and Lily Ling, when the cultures and relationships that form us are violent, this violence does not remain external to our selves.[3] Instead, it becomes integral to our identities. More specifically, human beings internalize patterns of thinking and acting that are rooted in the violence we experience through our interactions with culture and other people. This, in turn, shapes our actions and attitudes toward others and ourselves. For example, some who are subject to hate speech internalize negative self-images and a sense of alienation and despair. Others who survive a physical assault relive this violence in nightmares and flashbacks that recur repeatedly and against their will; they continue to hold within them the reality of the violence as ever present, even as they move through time.

In this book I develop a reconceptualization of Christian nonviolence that aims to address the problem of internal violence and to show how it can deepen traditional Christian views of nonviolence. In focusing on external violence, traditional views have explored the ways in which people and communities can act as *agents* of violence by performing actions that harm others or themselves. Recent accounts of internal violence, however, indicate that persons and communities also can become *sites* of violence as the violence they have experienced is incorporated into their identities. This raises the questions: How can Christian communities enact an alternative to violence when the church and its members are formed in and through violent cultures and relationships? What theological and practical resources might enable them to take part in transforming this violence, even as they are themselves constructed in a violent world? What, precisely, does it mean to enact nonviolence in relation to internal violence?

An integral part of my argument is that enacting nonviolence in relation to internal violence entails fostering the healing of individuals and communities that have been harmed by violence. In the pages ahead I explore, in conversation with both theological and theoretical sources, how Christian communities might embody this dimension of nonviolence in their life and worship. Theologically, Yoder serves as my primary conversation partner.[4] His work presents not only a view of nonviolence that I seek to challenge and deepen, but also a framework that contains useful resources for reconceptualizing nonviolence. Theoretically, I am in dialogue with two fields of study. First, feminist theory's descriptions of the self as deeply (though not necessarily entirely) socially constructed provide a conceptual basis for analyzing internal violence by highlighting ways in which people are formed in and through social contexts.[5]

Second, the interdisciplinary field of trauma studies vividly describes an acute form of violence that can become internal to the self over time: traumatic violence. Comprised of scholars and clinicians from many disciplines who all address "trauma" or "traumatic violence"—violence that leads to patterns of psychic wounding—this field analyzes a range of events and experiences. Some examples include war, sexual assault, domestic violence, and natural disasters. While those who study trauma do not use the language of "internal violence," it is precisely this dimension of violence that they address when describing trauma's ongoing effects. Trauma scholars understand trauma as a form of violence that can invade the self, breaking it down over time. For example, they contend that many survivors of one-time or repeated traumas remain haunted by these events long after they have passed, reliving them in nightmares, intrusive memories, and flashbacks. In these ways and more, trauma can become embedded in survivors' bodies, minds, and souls, causing them to experience this violence as an ongoing reality.

By exploring how trauma can become internalized over time, trauma scholars address a dimension of violence that Christian theologians often overlook. Many peace church theologians focus on war and state violence. Other theologians explore the physical violence that takes place in some churches, such as in cases of clergy sexual abuse.[6] From a different perspective, feminist and liberation theologians examine systemic violence by analyzing the institutions, social and liturgical practices, and political structures that harm particular groups of persons.[7] In contrast, trauma scholars focus on the self as a site of specific acts of harm. Rather than concentrating on the violence of institutions or macrostructures, they explore how violent traumatic acts can fragment persons over time, and how these individuals can (or cannot) heal from trauma's ongoing effects.

This emphasis on the individual self as a site of harm does not preclude analysis of social, institutional, and political structures and practices. Some trauma scholars emphasize the importance of analyzing structural harms by arguing that systems of oppression contribute to the perpetration of violent traumatic acts by creating conditions that sanction, support, and sustain this violence.[8] However, the structural dimensions of trauma are not the focus of trauma studies, particularly the Western psychological models that form the cornerstone of this field. Some criticize these models for precisely this reason. They argue that despite the enormous contributions that Western frameworks have made to our understanding of trauma's effects on individuals, these frameworks have a significant limitation: In focusing on the psychological aftermath of trauma, they sometimes portray trauma's lasting effects as an individual pathology rather than as partly the result of social injustices. Recently, several feminist trauma scholars have argued that this approach stigmatizes survivors and deflects attention from the real problem: the perpetrators of violence and the sociopolitical contexts that make trauma more likely to occur.[9]

In this book I offer descriptions of trauma and healing that attempt to address this potential limitation. To this end, I give an account of trauma and its effects that highlights not only its impact on individuals, but also the role that social and cultural contexts play in perpetrating violence and facilitating (or hindering) healing. The most significant way I do this is by paying attention to trauma studies' view of the self as fundamentally social and relational. By taking seriously the self's social character, one can counter the tendency to decontextualize trauma and its effects.

In taking into account the social and structural dimensions of trauma, however, my analysis does not extend to the broader societal or national level. This book does rely primarily on Western psychological frameworks for understanding trauma, and it therefore focuses on the "micro" rather than the "macro" level. Put simply, I consider how persons (and communities) can heal from trauma's effects, but do not explore what it takes to foster the recovery of an entire nation that has experienced trauma—such as Rwanda, Bosnia, or South Africa. While examining ways to reconstitute nations is vital, it opens up different issues from the ones I explore here. For example, it raises questions about how to rebuild political and economic infrastructures that war and mass violence have destroyed, how to reconcile ethnic groups whose histories are marked by political violence or genocide, and how to educate future generations so that collective violence does not happen again.

The smaller or "micro"-level questions addressed in this book shed light on a crucial matter for Christian communities: how they can provide a context where traumatized persons may heal from trauma's ongoing effects. This is an important matter to explore because trauma affects a large number of people and its impact is often severe. Many of the church's members are, in fact, trauma survivors. Moreover, some trauma scholars argue that trauma does not affect only those who have directly experienced it.[10] As people hear stories about others' traumas, they sometimes experience effects similar to those of the survivors, though to a lesser degree. This means that trauma can have an impact not just on some individuals in the church but on whole Christian communities.

From a theological perspective, one can ground this claim in an understanding of the church as a mutually interdependent social organism or "social body." As Letty Russell observes, if the church is a body in which all members are related, then what affects one also affects the others.[11] Therefore, while people who have suffered traumas such as domestic violence or natural disasters are affected by these events differently than those who have not, the problem of trauma is one with which the entire social body must contend. The nonviolence that the church is called to enact in relation to this violence is thus not something a few people can do on their own. It is a communal enterprise that requires the embodied participation of all those who constitute the church.

In exploring this dimension of nonviolence, it is important not to overestimate the power of Christian communities to assist traumatized persons or the extent to which they actually do so. As we will see in the pages ahead, some trauma survivors who look to Christian communities for help after their traumas do not find it there. Others report that the church has contributed to their healing, but acknowledge that they have found secular resources more beneficial. Moreover, churches throughout history have often perpetrated violence against their own members or those outside of their communities. The vision of nonviolence outlined in this book, therefore, describes not what Christian communities always do but something they are called to do. But while this vision is not fully embodied in present-day Christian communities, is also not entirely removed from them. Faith communities, despite their brokenness, can (and sometimes do) contribute to the healing of traumatized persons. The view of nonviolence that I offer here is thus "already" and "not yet" embodied in the concrete, historical realities of Christian communities.

In exploring this already and not yet in the life of the church, I consider ways in which theology and trauma studies can inform each other. On one level, I seek to discern how trauma can challenge and deepen our understanding of a central aspect of ecclesiology: the church's identity and mission. To that end, I bring the works of trauma scholars into conversation with theological topics relevant to discussions of trauma and its healing, such as the human person, the work of Jesus, and the kingdom of God. As I bring trauma studies into conversation with these classical themes of Christian theology, I explore how it can enrich theological discourse and provide new ways of thinking about the church's narratives, traditions, beliefs, and practices.

At the same time, the analysis in this book brings to light one important way in which these theological reflections on healing from trauma differ from the theoretical ones that many trauma scholars offer. As we will see, those who study trauma often argue that healing involves the reconstitution of the traumatized person's identity. In their view, the individual's identity is reconstituted through the love and support of communities that embody healthy, empowering relationships. In contrast, the theological account of healing that I develop in the pages ahead proposes that individuals also can heal—or have their identities re-formed—through their participation in the construction of a communal identity. Christians have both an individual identity and a communal identity as part of the body of Christ, and understanding the dynamic interplay between these two realities remains integral to discerning the church's possible role in assisting trauma survivors.

This book is not the first to put Christian theology and trauma studies in dialogue. Flora Keshgegian has drawn on the insights of trauma studies to explore how Christian communities can engage in the work of remembering in ways that both foster healing for trauma survivors and redeem Christianity from its own complicity in violence and oppression.[12] Jennifer Beste has examined how the findings of trauma studies challenge theological beliefs about human freedom and God's grace.[13] And in the immediate aftermath of 9/11, Serene Jones engaged trauma studies as a resource for analyzing the psychological effects of terrorism on our nation and for suggesting possible ways for Christian communities to respond.[14] These works all make important contributions to our understandings of theology, violence, and the human person. In this book I strive to continue this conversation by drawing on trauma studies to develop a new understanding of Christian nonviolence that addresses the often-overlooked reality of internal violence.

An outline of the book will indicate how the field of trauma studies is helpful in this task. But first I want to offer a brief note about terminology. I often refer to the multiplicity of Christian communities in the world as simply "the church." I do so not to deny their multiplicity and the many differences that distinguish these communities from each other, but to underscore that in the midst of their manyness, Christian communities are united. Theologians often use the phrase "the church" to suggest that all Christian communities are linked through their shared union with Christ's heavenly body, which takes place through the power of the Holy Spirit. Although these communities have differences and sometimes exist in conflict, we can, from a theological perspective, still refer to them as one body called "the church" or the "Christian community."

OUTLINE OF THE BOOK

Chapter 1 analyzes Yoder's understanding of nonviolence and its basis in the particular narratives of the life, death, and resurrection of Jesus. By exploring his interpretation of these biblical narratives, this analysis both lays out a conception of nonviolence that I seek to deepen and highlights theological resources that are useful for developing a redefinition of nonviolence in the later chapters. This assessment of Yoder's work also brings into focus the reality of internal or internalized violence, a dimension of violence that his writings on nonviolence do not explicitly address.

The second chapter considers traumatic violence as a particularly acute form of violence that can become internal to the self. In doing so, it illuminates the multiple ways that trauma can shatter the self as it moves from the outside in and becomes incorporated into one's identity. This description of trauma's effects indicates that nonviolence must go beyond pacifism and the refusal of external, physical violence to include the creation of communities in which traumatized persons can heal from the ongoing effects of traumatic violence. Chapter 3 then lays the theoretical foundation for discerning how churches might constitute such communities. It does so by exploring three steps that many trauma scholars consider necessary for healing or reconstituting traumatized persons: establishing safety, narrating the trauma, and "retemporalizing" the survivor.

The final three chapters develop a contemporary understanding of nonviolence by theologically reflecting on these phases of the healing process. Each chapter explores a correlation between Yoder's theology and trauma studies' accounts of recovery. Chapter 4 examines how Yoder's view of ecclesial relations both resonates with, and is challenged by, trauma studies' descriptions of supportive relationships. Chapter 5 considers parallels between Yoder's use of narrative and the role that many trauma scholars believe narrative plays in the healing process. Chapter 6 then explores Yoder's understanding of the church as an eschatological community in light of many trauma survivors' struggles to reconnect with the present and envision a better future. Taken together, these chapters redefine nonviolence to include the transformation of internalized, traumatic violence through the communal creation of a new identity.

These last three chapters are more reflective than prescriptive. This is not a "how to" manual for Christian communities, a guideline or set of specific recommendations for particular activities that Christian communities should perform to better assist trauma survivors. Instead, these chapters explore how faith communities already function, in some instances, as sources of support through their ordinary life and worship. While there are, no doubt, new measures that churches could implement which would benefit trauma survivors, they are not the focus of this book. Rather, this book theologically reflects on aspects of the Christian tradition's narratives and practices that enable some survivors to experience, perhaps in just small ways, healing from trauma.

One could undertake similar analysis in relation to other religious traditions, which each have their own resources. My choice to focus on the Christian traditions does not reflect an attempt to privilege Christianity over other religions. Rather, it simply indicates my desire to understand more fully what it means for Christian communities to live into their identities as nonviolent communities of faith. The stakes for them to do so are high; as we will see, when communities facilitate the healing of trauma survivors, they effect change in the world that extends beyond the lives of these individuals. When people develop the internal strength that comes with recovery from trauma, they often become empowered and motivated to actively participate in broader movements for change. Moreover, the healing of individuals and their communities is itself part of transformation of the world. Thus, when the church creates a context in which traumatized persons can survive and flourish, it enacts a powerful dimension of nonviolence, one that is much-needed in a world where violence has so many different forms and inspires such widespread terror. The church participates in the construction of communities and persons who become not only sites of violence, but also sites of grace.

NOTES

1. See Anne Llewellyn Barstown, "Nonviolent Interventions: A Response to Terrorism," *Church and Society* 94, no. 5 (May–June 2004): 25–33; David Cortright, *Gandhi and Beyond: Nonviolence for an Age of Terrorism* (Boulder, CO: Paradigm Publishers, 2006); Stephen A. Graham, "What Would Jesus Do about Terrorism? Christian Realism vs. Christian Pacifism," *Encounter* 65, no. 4 (Autumn 2004): 345–71; Tom H. Hastings, *Nonviolent Response to Terrorism* (Jefferson, NC: McFarland & Company, 2004); James L. Rowell, "Has Nonviolent Religion Been Trumped?" *Theology Today* 63, no. 2 (July 2006): 223–26; and Jim Wallis, "Hard Questions for Peace-

makers: Theologians of Nonviolence Wrestle with How to Resist Terrorism," *Sojourners Magazine* 31, no. 1 (January–February 2002): 29–33.

2. J. Denny Weaver, "Theology in the Mirror of the Martyred and Oppressed," *Wisdom of the Cross* (Grand Rapids, MI: Eerdmans, 1999), 424.

3. See bell hooks, *Sisters of the Yam: Black Women and Self-Recovery* (Boston: South End Press, 1993). For a brief discussion of internal violence and its challenge to traditional conceptions of nonviolence, see also Lisa Adler and L. H. M. Ling, "From Practice to Theory: Toward a Dissident-Feminist Reconstruction of Nonviolence," *Gandhi Marg: Journal of the Gandhi Peace Foundation*, 16, no. 4 (January–March 1995): 462–80.

4. In the course of writing this book, I came across an article that told of Yoder's sexual offenses against multiple women in the Mennonite community and the Mennonite church's subsequent decision to suspend his ministerial credentials ("Yoder Suspended," *Christian Century* 109, no. 24 (August 12, 1992): 737. Yoder's abusive actions may make it seem problematic to use his work as a constructive resource for a project on trauma and nonviolence. At the same time, I find his theological insights about discipleship and Christian community helpful for reconceptualizing nonviolence, even though he did not always embody these insights in his own life. My use of his work, then, is not intended to ignore or justify his actions, but rather to probe the possibilities of his ideas for developing a contemporary understanding of nonviolence.

5. In engaging constructivist understandings of the self and speaking of the self (and the community) as a "site," I am not endorsing certain postmodernist views of the self as utterly lacking in coherence or stability. The scholars whose work I draw on speak in ways which suggest that the self does have a core comprised of certain features, such as agency, relationality, memory, and embodiment. These capacities lend it an integrity or wholeness, even as it is marked by inevitable fissures.

6. For example, see Marie M. Fortune, *Is Nothing Sacred? When Sex Invades the Pastoral Relationship* (San Francisco: Harper & Row, 1989); Marie M. Fortune and James N. Poling, *Sexual Abuse by Clergy: A Crisis for the Church* (Decatur, GA: Journal of Pastoral Care Publications, 1994); and Nancy Hopkins Myer and Mark Laaser, *Restoring the Soul of a Church: Healing Congregations Wounded by Clergy Sexual Misconduct* (Washington, DC: Alban Institute, 1995).

7. For example, see Gustavo Gutierrez, *A Theology of Liberation: History, Politics, and Salvation*, translated and edited by Sister Caridad Inda and John Eagleson (Maryknoll, NY: Orbis Books, 1973, reprinted 1988); Serene Jones, *Feminist Theory and Christian Theology: Cartographies of Grace* (Minneapolis: Fortress Press, 2000); and Catherine Mowry LaCugna, ed., *Freeing Theology: The Essentials of Theology in Feminist Perspective* (New York: HarperCollins, 1993).

8. For example, see Laura S. Brown, "Not Outside the Range: One Feminist Perspective on Psychic Trauma," in *Trauma: Explorations in Memory*, ed. Cathy Caruth (Baltimore: Johns Hopkins University Press, 1995), 110–12; Mary E. Gilfus, "The Price of a Ticket: A Survivor-Centered Appraisal of Trauma Theory," *Violence Against Women* 5, no. 11 (November 1999): 1238–57; and Maria P. P. Root, "Reconstructing the Impact of Trauma on Personality," in *Personality and Psychopathology: Feminist Reappraisals*, eds. Laura S. Brown and Mary Ballou (New York: The Guilford Press, 1992), 229–61.

9. See Brown, "Not Outside the Range," Gilfus, "The Price of a Ticket," and Root, "Reconstructing the Impact of Trauma on Personality." My own analysis follows the example of clinical trauma studies in focusing on trauma survivors rather than trauma perpetrators. While the study of perpetrators is important, it opens up a different set of questions and concerns than the ones I address here.

10. See Brown, "Not Outside the Range," and Root, "Reconstructing the Impact of Trauma on Personality."

11. Letty M. Russell, Flora Keshgegian, *The Church with AIDS: Renewal in the Midst of Crisis,* ed. Letty M. Russell (Louisville, KY: Westminster John Knox Press, 1990), 26.

12. *Redeeming Memories: A Theology of Healing and Transformation* (Nashville, TN: Abingdon Press, 2000).

13. Jennifer Beste, *God and the Victim: Traumatic Intrusions on Grace and Freedom* (New York: Oxford University Press, 2007).

14. Serene Jones, "Emmaus Witnessing: Trauma and the Disordering of the Theological Imagination," *Union Seminary Quarterly Review* 55 no. 3–4 (2001): 113–28.

1

Nonviolence in the Theology of John Howard Yoder

During my first year of divinity school, a friend placed a copy of John Howard Yoder's *The Politics of Jesus* in my hand. "You should read this," she said. "It's written by that Mennonite theologian, the guy who advocates for nonviolence. It's really wild!"

As I read and re-read Yoder's work over the next few years, I came to see the ways in which her description both accurately described and misconstrued elements of his theological contribution. No doubt, Yoder presents a vision of nonviolence that has influenced many Christians in North America. And as my friend's comment implied, his work has not been uncontroversial. Many scholars describe him as a provocative or appropriately unsettling thinker, one who poses an important challenge to the ways in which mainstream Christians think about questions of violence and the normativity of Jesus for their social and political witness.[1] Other critics are less generous and respond to Yoder's challenge by simply dismissing his work, portraying him as a representative of a radical type of Christianity that does not offer a viable option for mainstream Christians.

Still others, however, persuasively argue that this dismissal overlooks the fact that Yoder was a significant figure not only in twentieth-century Mennonite studies, but also in ecumenical discussions in Europe and North America for nearly fifty years. Though often described (as the words of my friend indicate) as a Mennonite theologian, Yoder saw himself as one who wrote not only for the historic peace churches but for a broader Christian audience.[2] He sought to appeal to this audience by grounding his work in a story all Christians hold in common: the narratives of Jesus.[3] While some may contest his reading of scripture, Yoder himself saw his appeal to the Jesus story as an ecumenical position that he hoped would foster dialogue across the many Christian traditions.

Yoder's interpretation of the gospel narratives makes him stand out among contemporary theologians as one who articulates a view of Christian faith and discipleship that places nonviolence at its center. In an era where many Christians, including some members of the historic peace churches, find nothing within Christianity to support a nonviolent way of life, Yoder's work poses a welcome and thoughtful challenge. In this chapter I examine his reading of the gospel narratives to introduce some theological resources—such as the cross, resurrection, and kingdom of God—that make important contributions to Christian understandings of nonviolence.

At the same time, the examination of Yoder's work in this chapter provides a vision of nonviolence that I seek to deepen in the latter stages of this book. Whereas Yoder focuses on how Christians can enact nonviolence in relation to violence that is external to their communities, I want to explore how the church can potentially transform violence that has become incorporated into the identities of Christian communities and those who constitute them. Yoder's interpretation of the life, death, and resurrection of Jesus, his view of discipleship, and his description of the nature of Christian community provide valuable resources for this exploration. I begin with his work, then, not to reject or embrace it but to open up a dialogue with his writings that ultimately seeks to illuminate a dimension of human existence he does not consider.

JESUS AND THE POLITICS OF CHRISTIAN NONVIOLENCE

When Yoder published his groundbreaking book *The Politics of Jesus* in 1972, many readers were stunned by the boldness of one of its central claims: Jesus is not only relevant but also *normative* for Christian social ethics. Throughout this text Yoder criticizes structures of ethical reasoning that turn away from the biblical narratives and refuse to see Jesus as the social-political-ethical standard for the Christian life. For him, these ways of thinking fail to take seriously the implications of the classical Christian affirmation that Jesus reveals the true nature and calling of humanity.[4] In Yoder's perspective, this claim implies that Jesus is normative for those who have made a confession of faith in him. This does not mean, however, that the church needs to imitate every aspect of his existence. Yoder argues that the New Testament does not indicate that Christians must take as a model "Jesus' trade as a carpenter, his association with fishermen, and his choice of illustrations from the life of the sower and the shepherd. . . ."[5] Rather, the gospels have a specific focus: "Only at one point, only on one subject—but then consistently, universally—is Jesus our example: in his cross."[6]

Yoder does not emphasize the cross of Jesus to endorse a theology of martyrdom or to glorify suffering. Rather, he means to say that the cross marks the culmination of a specific way of life: a life of nonviolence and social nonconformity in relation to the world's dominant social and political structures. As the summation of this way of life, the cross provides the lens through which we can interpret other aspects of Jesus' story. To suggest that Jesus is our example only in his cross, then, is to indicate that this event demonstrates most clearly his way of life, and we cannot understand these two aspects of his existence in isolation. In *The Politics of Jesus,* Yoder examines in detail Jesus' death and its meaning for Christian social ethics. He begins, however, not with the cross, but with an exploration of Jesus' life and ministry as described in the gospels.

Yoder draws primarily on the book of Luke to paint a picture of Jesus as a "radical rabbi" who establishes a new social reality.[7] In his view, these biblical texts show that Jesus set out to construct a voluntary and egalitarian society of mixed composition in which all persons live together in peace.[8] For Yoder, Jesus' creation of this new human community is a response to both Israel's experience of Roman occupation and Zealot revolutions. Jesus was a "displaced person in a foreign occupation and puppet governments" who had to choose among several ways of dealing with the social conflict he encountered.[9] Yoder asserts that he rejected the revolutionary violence of the Zealots, the passivity of the Herodians and Sadducees, and the social withdrawal of the Pharisees. Jesus selected instead a different option: the formation of a distinct, covenanting community that embodies a specific way of life.[10]

For Yoder, one distinguishing feature of Jesus' life is his refusal to use the political power and revolutionary violence at his disposal. In his life and ministry, Jesus consistently rejects the temptation to seize the kingship and the kind of power offered him, which is the power to rule society and to govern the course of history. For example, in the temptations that Jesus experiences in the wilderness before his public ministry, he is presented with the possibility of using power to take over and direct all the kingdoms of the world—an offer he turns down.[11] Similarly, when he later realizes that the five thousand people he has just fed from five loaves and two fish are about to make him king, Jesus withdraws from the crowd and goes to the mountain by himself. [12]

Yoder argues that in rejecting this power, Jesus does not reject power itself. Instead, he chooses to use a different kind of power. Jesus elects not to rule but to serve, and "servanthood is not a position of nonpower or weakness. It is an alternative mode of power . . . a way to make things happen."[13] Yoder's reading of the gospel narratives of the cross supports this claim. He notes that after Peter confesses Jesus as the messiah, Jesus does not withdraw from the crowd and retreat into the wilderness. Instead, he goes to Jerusalem, the center of Jewish and Roman power. Yoder writes that

> what he proposes is not withdrawal into the desert or into mysticism; it is a renewed messianic claim, a mountaintop consultation with Moses and Elijah, and a march to Jerusalem. The cross is beginning to loom not as a ritually prescribed instrument of propitiation but as the political alternative to both insurrection and quietism.[14]

For Yoder, the cross is a political alternative to insurrection because it reveals Jesus' refusal to conquer his enemies with force. It offers a political alternative to quietism because it directly confronts the authorities who ultimately kill him.[15]

In describing the cross as a *political* option, Yoder challenges the assumption that nonviolence is a-political. His argument depends on a particular conception of politics. For Yoder, politics does not simply refer to matters pertaining to the state and its government. The Greek word *polis* is often translated as "city," but it does not refer merely to the buildings in a specific geographical area or to the people who populate this space.[16] Rather, the word *polis* refers to "the orderly way in which [people] live together and make decisions, the way they structure their common life."[17] Thus, "To be political is to make decisions, to assign roles, and to distribute powers . . . 'Politics' affirms an unblinking recognition that we deal with matters of power, of rank and of money, of costly decisions and dirty hands, of memories and feelings."[18] On this definition, the life and death of Jesus represent a political alternative insofar as they reveal one way of dealing with the power wielded by the authorities of his day: the way of nonviolence.

Yoder notes that most accounts of politics would view the nonviolent politics of Jesus as a failure, since he appears not to triumph over his adversaries but rather dies a public and humiliating death. But these understandings of politics err, partly because they assume that immediate effectiveness is the goal. The politics of the cross rests on a different way of thinking, one that assumes neither that the relationship between cause and effect remains visible, nor that human beings are sufficiently informed "to be able to set for ourselves and for all society the goal toward which we seek to move it."[19]

The politics of the cross assumes that faithfulness to Jesus is what is ultimately effective, and the normal path of this faithfulness involves brokenness and suffering, the price of living a life of social nonconformity in relation to society's dominant social and political structures. Christians, therefore, must make their ethical decisions not on the basis of what they think they can accomplish immediately but on the basis of Jesus' example. Yoder notes that this does not mean that Christians should give up analyzing how the world's systems work and how they can best contribute to changing them. They must continue to care about social analysis, but they must temper this analysis with the belief that Jesus reveals God's will and sets the standard for how history is moved.[20]

Even as Yoder argues that the church's nonviolence is based on obedience to Jesus rather than an estimation of immediate success, he refuses to give up on the efficacy of this way of life. He believes that the church's nonviolence will provide, in the long run, the best way to achieve social change. When Christians base their ethics on the example of Jesus, their efforts are guaranteed to "work"—not because of their own power but because God's resurrection power that raised Jesus from the dead has affirmed this as the appropriate way of life for his followers. For Yoder, "The relationship between the obedience of God's people and the triumph of God's cause is not a relationship of cause and effect but one of cross and resurrection."[21] Christians can be sure that embodying the way of Jesus ultimately will transform unjust social relations and structures because this way of life has its roots in the cross, which itself was an effective political stance (as confirmed by the resurrection). To understand in what sense Yoder considers the way of the cross a political stance that can lead to social change, and how it can make a difference in the world for Christians to embody this stance, it is helpful to consider his analysis of the cross and the problem Jesus confronts in this event: sin and evil.

RESISTING THE POWERS AND PRINCIPALITIES

When Yoder talks about sin and evil, he focuses not on the acts of individuals but on the powers and principalities. In his discussion on "Christ and Power," Yoder observes that the biblical language of power is ambiguous and unsystematic, primarily because Paul applies it to different challenges in different situations.[22] Rather than seeking to clarify this ambiguity by offering a succinct definition of the powers, he makes the general claim that they are that which bring order and regularity to God's good creation. The powers can be understood as what today we would call power structures—the state, institutions, and so on—but they cannot be simply reduced to this, for they are intangible as well. If this explanation seems somewhat unclear, Yoder sheds further light on the character of the powers by delineating two important facts about them: God created them for the purpose of ordering human existence, and they have both visible and invisible, material and spiritual forms.[23]

Having outlined the basic characteristics of the powers, Yoder describes their complex role in relation to humanity. He asserts that we need the powers to keep our world running smoothly. Human society, history, and even nature require regularity and order, and God has created the powers for this purpose.[24] But like the rest of God's creatures, the powers have rebelled and are fallen. In their fallenness, they seek to separate us from God's love by demanding that we adhere to values opposed to God's will. The powers now "[hold] us in servitude to their rules . . . . These structures which were supposed to be our servants have become our masters and our guardians."[25] Human beings are bound to the powers. This means we are enslaved to the values and structures that are essential for ordering human social life but that have "succeeded in making us serve them as if they were of absolute value."[26] This, in Yoder's view, describes our fallenness, our lost condition outside of Jesus.

Since human beings are enslaved to the powers, Jesus' work must involve liberating us from the powers' control. Yoder begins to explain this process of liberation by stating that even in their rebelliousness, the powers remain under God's providential sovereignty. God still uses them for God's creative purpose. Thus,

> Subordination to these Powers is what makes us human, for if they did not exist there would be no history nor society nor humanity. If then God is going to save his creatures *in their humanity*, the Powers cannot simply be destroyed or set aside or ignored. Their sovereignty must be broken. This is what Jesus did, concretely and historically, by living a genuinely free and human existence. This life brought him, as any genuinely human existence will bring anyone, to the cross.[27]

Since the powers are God's creatures and are necessary for ordering human society, we must not attempt to obliterate them. But since they are fallen, we must resist them. Jesus reveals the form this resistance should take in his life and death, when he defeats (but does not destroy) the powers by "subordinating" himself to their control, by declining to use the power at his disposal to crush them. This refusal to overwhelm his adversaries with sheer force is an act of resistance because it means that Jesus has not allowed the powers to make him over in their image. He has lived in their midst without becoming enslaved to their violent and self-serving ways.

How, then, does Jesus' subordination to the powers defeat them? Yoder views Jesus' death on the cross as an effective political action that defeats the powers by exposing their violent truth and thereby disarming them. To explain how the powers are exposed and disarmed, he cites Hendrikus Berkhof's claim that Jesus "made a public example of them."[28] Before God became incarnate in Jesus, the powers were seen as the true rulers of the world; through Jesus' work on earth, it became clear that the powers are against God's purposes. Jesus willingly subordinated himself to the powers and morally contradicted their values "by refusing to support them in their self-glorification; and that is why they killed him."[29] By existing in the midst of the powers but refusing to be enslaved by them, he provoked the powers to reveal that they work against God rather than in accord with God's will.[30] This revelation that the powers oppose God is their disarming, their defeat at the hands of Jesus. However, that Jesus not only opposes the powers but also triumphs over them can be known only in light of the resurrection, which manifests his victory on the cross. The resurrection reveals that at the cross, God has challenged the powers and demonstrated that God is stronger than they are.[31]

For Yoder, the resurrection not only manifests the victory that takes place on the cross, but also confirms God's approval of nonviolence as a way of life for Jesus and his disciples. It does so by disclosing the pattern of God's activity in the world as a whole: "'cross and resurrection' designates not only a few days' events in first-century Jerusalem but also the shape of the cosmos."[32] The resurrection means that God's redeeming Spirit is at work in the world and that through this Spirit people can have present-day experiences of transformation and renewal, even where there seems to be no reason for hope. It thus affirms what the cross, left on its own, would call into question: that God remains in control of history and will find a way to work things out, although human beings cannot see how this is possible.[33] In light of the resurrection, then, Christians can live according to the way of the cross with confidence that their actions will be vindicated in the end, even though in the present time they cannot see precisely how.

One reason many Christians find it difficult to believe that their faithful actions ultimately will "work" is that even in the aftermath of Jesus' victory, the powers continue to have harmful consequences. For example, both the acts of violence that people perpetrate and the structural injustices of our society which harm individuals and groups are evidence of the powers' continued effects—evidence that seems to belie the claim that Jesus has triumphed over them. Since the powers still clearly have destructive force, Yoder argues that Jesus has defeated them *ultimately*; his work has challenged the powers' uncontested ability to convince human beings that they are the "divine regents" of the world.[34] But this ultimate defeat does not render the powers entirely impotent in the present. To use an eschatological image that theologians often draw on, Jesus' triumph is "already" and "not yet" manifest in history.

Though Yoder maintains that Jesus' death and resurrection have defeated the powers ultimately, he cautions that we cannot understand the full significance of Jesus' work without considering the close connection between the cross and the church. The work of Jesus does not end with his victory over the powers on the cross, but instead continues in the life of the Christian community. Since the powers still seek to control the existing social order, the church is called to show them that their unchallenged dominion has come to an end. It can do this by refusing to be seduced by the powers, by living as the new social humanity that Jesus created. Nonviolence and servanthood must, therefore, constitute the essence of the church's identity and witness. By incarnating this stance in its own life, the church manifests Jesus' victory—and in this way continues to undermine the potency of the powers by reminding them of their ultimate defeat.[35]

CHURCH AS AN ALTERNATIVE CONSTRUCTION OF THE WORLD

Yoder contends that when Christian communities embody the nonviolence and servanthood exemplified by Jesus of Nazareth, they manifest a certain difference from something called "the world." Often, he refers to the Christian community as "other" than the world, an "alternative community" or "alternative construction of the world."[36] At times he says that the church is called to be "against" the world, even as it is "in, with, and for" the world.[37] What, precisely, does Yoder mean when he makes these claims? How are we to understand the concepts of "world" and "otherness" in his work and their relation to Christian nonviolence?

Let's begin with "the world." For Yoder, "world" is a collective term for the powers and principalities—the material and spiritual structures instituted by God to order human society—that oppose the work of Jesus. More precisely, Yoder states that the world consists of those "acts and institutions that are by their nature—and not solely by an accident of context or motivation—denials of faith in Christ."[38] Thus, he does not view the world as all of culture or society. Rather, he understands it as culture that is "*self-glorifying* or culture *as autonomous* and rebellious and oppressive, opposed to authentic human flourishing."[39] In Yoder's perspective, the world is not wholly evil, for the powers of the world continue to provide order and regularity, even in their fallenness. He writes, "The 'world' of politics, the 'world' of economics, the 'world' of the theater, the 'world' of sports . . . each is a demonic blend of order and revolt."[40]

In defining the world in this way, Yoder indicates that the basic distinction between church and world is between belief and unbelief.[41] Unlike the world, the church consists of persons who have made a confession of faith in Jesus. By virtue of this confession, Christians are called to live as his faithful disciples. Yoder writes:

> The need is not . . . for most Christians to get out of the church and into the world. They have been in the world all the time. The trouble is that they have been *of* the world, too. The need is for what they do in the world to be different because they are Christian; to be a reflection not merely of their restored self-confidence nor of their power to set the course of society, but of the social novelty of the covenant of grace.[42]

As a community that has made a confession of faith in Jesus, the church must manifest its faith by reflecting the grace of God's reconciling or community-building love.

In describing Yoder's view of the church-world distinction, it is important to note that he does not say that the basis for this distinction is that the church is sinless, while the world is not. The church itself is a power or structure, [43] and it is therefore subject to corruption.[44] Yoder does allow for the possibility of moral growth in this life; he believes the church can facilitate this moral improvement by providing a context in which people can imagine and practice new patterns of thinking and relating.[45] But he also maintains a strong sense of the sinfulness of all persons and institutions.[46] Given this belief in the omnipresence of sin, he does not ask Christians for perfection. Instead, he asks that they strive to live in faithfulness to Jesus and to manifest his identity in the world, however imperfectly. Yoder's distinction between church and world is, therefore, not a distinction between perfect people and sinful people. On one level, it is a distinction between sinful people who confess faith in Jesus and commit to following after him, and sinful people who do not make such a confession and commitment.[47]

While Yoder recognizes the church's peccability, he holds out the possibility that it can respond creatively to the powers, in ways that follow the nonviolent example of Jesus.[48] His belief in the possibility of creative response to the powers is grounded in his conviction that Christians have "resources of faith," including the support of the Christian community, training in this community's discipleship lifestyle, the guidance of the Holy Spirit, and a regenerate will. Yoder thinks that as a result of these resources, the church can embody Jesus' way of nonviolence in the world, though never perfectly. There is brokenness in the church, but it can still be a "specifiably Christian" community that follows after Jesus and manifests his identity in the world.[49]

For Yoder, this specificity of the Christian community means that it must remain visible as a distinctive social body in the world. He suggests that while the Christian community is visible by its practices—such as baptism and breaking bread together—the real essence of its visibility is its manifestation of a new set of relationships, which these practices help to create and sustain. For Yoder, God's work is to bring into being a "new humanity" of social wholeness, in both the Old Covenant and the New.[50] As this new humanity, the church must embody relationships that differ from the ones often found in the wider society—egalitarian and reconciling relationships that disrupt social hierarchies and allow persons of various backgrounds and persuasions to live together in peace.

Yoder asserts that the visible character of the church is essential to its identity and mission, for at least two reasons. First, the church's mission, first and foremost, is to be the church, a faith community that embodies a specific set of relationships. However, the church cannot be this community if it identifies with the world's dominant social powers, which are hierarchically structured and thus create divisions between persons of different backgrounds. According to Yoder, if the church aligns itself with society's dominant powers, then it will remain unable to foster a community of diverse people.[51]

Second, Yoder says that the church has a mission to engage in meaningful evangelism in the world, and it can do this only if it constitutes a community that embodies the way of life that it hopes others will likewise embrace.[52] Though this observation makes a practical point, Yoder asserts that it goes beyond mere pragmatism and gets to the heart of the gospel itself. In his view, the gospel says that the work of Jesus is, in part, to create a new social humanity which brings together different people in relationships of interdependence, reciprocal accountability, and mutual empowerment.[53] The distinctness or visibility of the church is, therefore, a *"prerequisite to the meaningfulness of the gospel message."*[54]

In describing the church as this "new humanity" that is other than the world, Yoder asserts that the world is not a "tangible, definable quantity" that simply sits over-against the church.[55] Rather, several points of connection between church and world exist. For example, Yoder says that the church is linked to the world by the fact that it is called to serve the world as an agent of positive change.[56] He further notes that church and world are de-polarized[57] when the world's powers are limited and made useful, thanks to the work of Jesus and to the church that continues his ministry.[58] In his view, Christians should not be optimistic about the good the powers can do, or about what they can accomplish by working with and through these powers.[59] Nonetheless, there are times and places in which the church's ministry or the workings of Providence do divest the powers of their destructiveness so that they can be used for good purposes.[60] If the powers sometimes are tamed, then it is too simplistic simply to say that the world constitutes an evil system that stands entirely apart from the church.[61]

Yoder also indicates that the church and world are related by the world's presence in Christians' individual and social lives.[62] As fallen form of creation, the world is unbelief; and those who profess faith in Jesus participate in this unbelief as well. Put differently, Yoder recognizes that people's lives are a mixture of belief and unbelief; institutions, too, are a "blend of order and revolt."[63] In light of this complex relation between church and world, belief and unbelief, he advocates not "the creation, over against the world, of a 'church' that just sits there at odds with the world, but rather an ongoing critical process."[64] This critical process requires the church to discern which aspects of the world it must reject and which it can accept. It also requires the church to criticize its own identity.[65] Since the Christian community manifests unbelief as well as belief, it must always seek to improve its faithfulness by analyzing the ways in which it is failing to live into its identity as the new humanity that God has brought into being.

In exploring how the church can live more faithfully into its identity, Yoder does not assert that only the Christian community can embody an ethical stance similar to the one manifested by Jesus. At times he insists that the language of "visibility," "distinctiveness," and "otherness" does not necessarily imply that the church embodies a clear ethical difference from other communities in the wider culture that object to violence and injustice. Sometimes, what makes Christian communities "specific" or "distinctive" is not what they do, but the reasons they do it or their willingness to continue when their actions appear not to be "working."[66] Yoder's discussion of the church-world distinction thus does not set the church apart as the sole community that can incarnate a set of values and relationships that differ from what one commonly finds in the broader culture. It does, however, suggest that the Christian community is the only one that would embody these values and relationships based on faith in Jesus.

Often, Yoder's critics take his insistence that the church must live as the new social humanity Jesus created as evidence that he thinks the church should enact an ethic of withdrawal, living as a "sect" on the margins of society and remaining unconcerned with the problems of the world. Yoder, however, contends that this is not the case. Conformity to the way of Jesus does not imply a lack of concern for the current social order. Quite the opposite is true: The nonviolent church must remain an active presence within society, struggling to achieve positive social change. Put differently, Yoder asserts that even as the Christian community is called to be "other" than or "against" the world, it must be, at the same time, "in" and "for" the world. His construal of the relationship between ecclesiology and social ethics clarifies this perplexing claim and illuminates how he thinks nonviolent communities can bring about genuine social change.

THE SOCIAL ETHICS OF THE ALTERNATIVE COMMUNITY

Yoder's understanding of the relationship between ecclesiology and social ethics rests on a central claim: The church does not first become a faith community and then enact a particular social ethic. Rather, the church's living as the new humanity created by the work of God is itself a social ethic. Yoder underscores the inseparability of the church's social shape and the substance of its social ethics when he writes, "peoplehood and mission, fellowship and witness, are not two desiderata, each capable of existing or of being missed independently of one another; each is the condition of the genuineness of the other."[67] In the very processing of becoming a faith community that does certain things together, the church engages the broader society. Yoder explains, "To participate in the transforming process of becoming the faith community *is itself* to speak the prophetic word, *is itself* the beginning of the transformation of the cosmos."[68]

Yoder's account of the powers and principalities clarifies how he thinks the church can have a transforming impact on the wider society simply by being the church. As David Toole observes, Yoder indicates that the church, by being a new social humanity in the middle of the current social order, incarnates a "concrete rearrangement" of this order and thereby begins to restructure its power relations. This restructuring of power relations, in Yoder's view, is itself an act of resistance to society's unjust social relations and structures. The notion that restructuring power relations is an act of resistance depends on the idea that the powers are part of God's good creation. As noted above, Yoder argues that since the powers are part of God's creation, Christians must not destroy them through frontal assault. The church's task is rather to show them that their rebellion has been overcome in Jesus by living as a community that remains freed from their destructive ways.[69] Here, he is suggesting that the new covenantal rule within the church can rupture the hierarchical character of the powers and, without making a direct assault upon them, subvert and transform them. The church's formation of a community that enacts the stance of Jesus thus can be the first step in a process of significant social change, though one cannot always account for exactly how that change takes place.

In addition to this somewhat obscure account of how the church can participate in the transformation of the current social order, Yoder gives several concrete explanations. First, he suggests that the church, simply by being a new kind of community that remains present on the social scene, can provide an example for the world to follow. The church can model for the world an alternative way of making decisions (through open dialogue and consensus).[70] It can also show the world how to feed the hungry and care for the sick.[71] By setting such examples, the church can influence the world through "moral osmosis,"[72] making an indirect contribution "to the development of generally recognized moral standards" outside of the Christian community.[73] Though the church cannot expect the world to adhere to the same degree of love, forgiveness, and nonviolence to which the church is called, it can show the world how to live in a more loving and forgiving and less violent way. For example, Yoder observes that Christian organizations performed international relief work for victims of war and natural disasters before governments became involved in such efforts. Similarly, the church provided the services of schools and hospitals before the larger society began to manage such institutions.[74]

Yoder also asserts that the church can serve the world by speaking directly to it. The fact that the church is called to be a nonviolent community that is "other" than the world does not mean that it should not address the world if it has something to say.[75] In speaking to the world, the Christian community can lobby its institutions and agencies, though it should not be overly optimistic about the chances of immediate success.[76] Yoder claims, "The world can be challenged, at the most, on one point at a time, to take one step in the right direction, to approximate in a slightly greater degree the righteousness of love."[77] One way to facilitate this communication between church and world is to use "middle axioms," principles that both parties hold and to which they are both accountable—such as the need to care for the poor and to show respect for human rights.[78] The existence of these middle axioms, in Yoder's view, enables Christians to offer a meaningful social critique that challenges the world to address and remedy specific injustices that occur in given times and places. This does not mean, however, that Christians may impose their ways on the social order. When it addresses the world, the church should embody a posture of humility, rather than one of domination.

For Yoder, the church's service to the world should also involve its active participation in opposing social injustice. Far from showing a lack of concern for society, he argues that "the love of a sovereign God drives [Christians] into concern for the social order."[79] Christians must identify and strive to transform oppressive social relations and structures, but they must remain committed to making these changes "*in the way of Christ.*"[80] For Yoder, this means that the church should strive to transform society through nonviolent ways of resisting injustice and oppression. In his view, Christians must take such service in and to the world quite seriously, for the life of discipleship may prove costly. Above all, then, the church must witness to the world through its deeds—even to the point of being willing to suffer for the sake of its faith.[81]

By emphasizing the active dimension of nonviolence, Yoder's work challenges those who would equate nonviolence with doing nothing. Often, critics of a nonviolent social ethic argue that nonviolence leads people to become passive in the face of evil, to simply stand by and watch while others suffer. Considering the immense horrors perpetrated daily around the world, such a response is understandably characterized as inadequate. Yoder, however, makes it clear that inaction is not what he advocates. He stresses that Christian nonviolence has a positive or creative dimension: It involves not just withdrawing from violence, but also striving to resist and transform specific injustices in the current social order.[82] In pointing to this positive dimension of nonviolence, Yoder indicates that the nonviolent church is not irrelevant to the social issues of its day. It does not ignore these issues, but rather directly engages them precisely by acting as a nonviolent agent of social change.

In developing this vision of the church, Yoder not only makes a compelling argument for nonviolence, but also challenges many Christians to rethink some of their fundamental theological beliefs and perceptions. Specifically, he calls into question the common tendency to dismiss Jesus as the true revelation of God's character and will. He likewise challenges the need human beings often have to feel that we are in control of the world and can direct the course of history. And he critically evaluates the assumption that immediate results are the measure of genuine success. In interrogating these basic convictions, Yoder points Christians toward an alternative way of thinking—one which asserts that the direction of history ultimately lies not in our hands but in the hands of God; that it is precisely when we try to control the world that we inevitably do the most damage; that there is more to the world than we can see with our own eyes; and that nonviolence may work in ways that we cannot recognize at the current time.

As we have seen, Yoder's confidence that nonviolence ultimately "works" stems not from abstract ideas about the incarnation or specific doctrines but from the biblical narratives of the life, death, and resurrection of Jesus. In chapter 5 I explore further the significance of his turn to these narratives, asking how "narrative" functions in his work and how the gospel narratives, in particular, might speak to those whose lives have been shattered by overwhelming violence. Though I move beyond Yoder's writings in these latter stages of the book, I have begun with his interpretation of the biblical narratives because it offers key resources for reconceptualizing nonviolence. Yoder's reading of Jesus' life and death, his account of the powers, and his understanding of Christian community and discipleship provide valuable tools for exploring a new dimension of nonviolence: the transformation or healing of the ongoing effects of violence.

INTERNAL VIOLENCE: THE SELF AS A SITE OF VIOLENCE

Yoder's work, however, does not provide the theoretical analysis of violence needed for this re-examination of nonviolence. His view of Christian nonviolence centers on pacifism and the refusal of military violence, which is not surprising, given that historically these have represented central concerns of Mennonite peace theology.[83] However, this understanding of nonviolence misses an important form of "violence." It addresses what some scholars call external violence, but it does not explicitly attend to the reality of internal violence.[84]

What, exactly, is the difference between external and internal violence? At a most basic level, external violence consists of violent harms that assault people from without.[85] Within this category, one can include acts of overt physical force perpetrated by one individual or group against another, such as when one person strikes another or when the police brutalized civil rights activists in the south during the 1950s and 1960s. In addition to such instances of physical aggression, external violence includes systemic forms of oppression, which are not necessarily overtly physical and are perpetrated through the social, economic and political structures of society. A concrete example is poverty, which restricts people's access to the basic necessities of human life.

In contrast to external violence, "internal" or "internalized" violence refers to violence that has assaulted people from without and then become embedded within their bodies, minds, and souls. For example, scholars and clinicians who study the long-term effects of physical violence often observe that many persons who have survived this violence relive it through nightmares, flashbacks, and intrusive memories that recur repeatedly and against their will.[86] In this way, they continue to experience the violence as held within them and ever present, even as they move through time. Along similar lines, internalized violence includes forms of systemic violence, such as sexism and racism, which not only harm us from without but also profoundly shape our ways of thinking and being in the world. For instance, some people who are repeatedly subjected to hate speech and other forms of degradation turn "inwards and against themselves," internalizing negative self-images and a profound sense of alienation and despair.[87]

One way to understand how violence becomes internalized is to consider the social construction of identity—or, in common parlance, the ways that "nurture" or "socialization" help make us who we are.[88] In recent years, it has become commonplace to say that human beings are shaped in and through our social, economic, political, and cultural contexts. While scholars hold differing views about how "deep" this social construction goes—some think we are more the products of our environment than others—those who endorse constructivism agree that our identities have a dynamic character: We develop and change as we encounter new cultural forces, events, discourses, and traditions that help constitute us into the unique persons we are.

This ongoing process of social formation is not itself violent. Human beings can, in fact, be formed in many nonviolent ways. However, violence does become integral to our identities when the relationships and cultures that form us are violent. For example, as we are shaped in and by a sexist, racist, and classist society, we learn to relate to others (and ourselves) in sexist, racist, and classist ways. In noting that violence can move into the self in these ways, it is important to stress that no one is immune from this harm. While we are not merely passive in our social formation, we all internalize violence (though not in the same ways and to the same degree), given our participation in a society in which violence is manifested in so many different forms.

In his famous "Letter from Birmingham Jail," Martin Luther King, Jr. gives a concrete example of how violence can become internalized through social construction. Addressing the eight white clergy who criticized his activism in Birmingham as unwise and untimely, King explains what racism does to the human mind and spirit. He describes a young black girl who learns that she cannot go to the public amusement park because it remains open only to whites. When she finds out why she can't go, "ominous clouds of inferiority" start to form "in her little mental sky . . . "[89] King further describes segregation as a system that instills in blacks a "degenerating sense of 'nobodiness.'"[90] Such examples indicate his awareness that violence does not remain external to those it violates (nor does it remain external to those who perpetrate the harm). Instead, it becomes internalized, shaping our psyches in a debilitating and deformative way.

This internalization of violence points to a second, related distinction that remains crucial for reconceptualizing nonviolence: the self as an "agent" of violence and the self as a "site" of violence. Traditional accounts of Christian nonviolence focus on ways in which people and communities can act as agents of violence by harming others or themselves. An analysis of internal violence, however, indicates that individuals (and communities) also can become sites of violence as the violence they have experienced is incorporated into their identities. Note that these categories of "agent" and "site" of violence are not mutually exclusive. Sometimes, our harmful actions and words are rooted in the violence that has become part of our own identities; the violence we have experienced and internalized becomes the space out of which we think and act. For example, King warns that the oppressed may find themselves tempted to engage in hate campaigns and physical violence against their oppressors.[91] Similarly, some scholars indicate that a small percentage of individuals who grow up in abusive homes commit violence against their own children or partners later in life.[92] Like external and internal violence, then, the self as agent and as site of violence are distinct but interrelated.

This distinction between the self as site and agent of violence points to the need to expand traditional Christian understandings of nonviolence. Rather than focusing only on how the church can resist external violence by refusing to act as an agent of violence, it is necessary to consider as well how it might contribute to the transformation of internal violence. As King's work suggests, this transformation remains integral to the creation of persons who have the wholeness that empowers them to participate in efforts to stop cycles of external violence in the world. A crucial dimension of nonviolence, then, is the healing of selves and communities that have been formed as sites of violence.

There exist at least two different kinds of violence that we can internalize through our social formation. First, as I have already suggested, human beings can internalize systemic violence by living in a world where we encounter violence as part of our daily lives, either as victims or oppressors (or both). For example, simply by living within a culture in which systemic violence is perpetrated in various ways—through degrading images in the media, discriminatory hiring practices, and cultural systems of value that exclude and stigmatize certain people—we internalize violence. As King indicates, this violence has a destabilizing or demoralizing force. For example, some individuals find that their sense of self is diminished, their confidence is undermined, and their voices are silenced.

At the same time, we have the power to resist systemic forms of violence in many ways. For example, one way we are constructed is through our consumption of representations and images that we encounter in the media.[93] But as consumers we are not simply dominated by these images against our will; we also choose much of what we consume. In addition to thoughtful selection, we can consume images with a certain awareness of their effects, a critical eye that mediates their impact on us.[94]

A second kind of violence, however, has a particularly destructive force when internalized. Traumatic violence—violence that leads to patterns of psychic wounding—represents an especially severe form of harm, one that not everyone experiences firsthand. For those who do, however, it can lead to psychological, physical, and spiritual symptoms that break down the self. For example, scholars and clinicians who study trauma observe that individuals who have traumatic experiences often suffer from intrusive flashbacks that make it difficult to concentrate, a loss of memory that renders them unable to recall specific events or whole periods of time, and a profound sense of depression and despair. Trauma thus represents a kind of "external" violence that can become embedded within (or "internal to") individuals in ways that not only destabilize them but also deeply fragment their identities over time.

This fragmentation calls into question one of Yoder's key assumptions about the human person. Yoder's vision of Christian nonviolence assumes that human beings have an agency that remains intact or whole. For example, his insistence that Christians can oppose the powers and principalities nonviolently is based partly on the conviction that, as a result of the Spirit's work, they are ontologically regenerate and thus have wills strong enough to resist the patterns of violence and injustice to which they have been exposed. Research studies on trauma, however, challenge the notion that all persons enjoy the wholeness or coherence that Yoder assumes. They suggest, using Yoder's terminology, that sometimes the violence of the powers can embed themselves so deeply in people that they experience a fracturing of their identities which makes it difficult to sustain the internal coherence necessary for living a life of Christian discipleship.

Contemporary understandings of Christian nonviolence need to take into account traumatic violence and explore how Christian communities can address the ongoing effects of this violence. In undertaking this exploration, it is important to emphasize that traumatic violence is not just an individual problem, something those whose lives have been shattered by trauma should strive to address on their own. In *The Church Has Aids*, Letty Russell argues that Christian communities are social organisms or social bodies in which what affects one affects all.[95] Thus, while individuals in the church who have directly experienced traumas such as domestic or sexual violence are affected by this violence differently than those who have not, the problem of trauma is one that has an impact on the entire community and therefore must be addressed by the church as a whole. Those who constitute the Christian community must struggle together with the questions: What does it mean for Christians to enact nonviolence when violence becomes integral to their individual and communal identities? How might one rethink the meaning and practice of nonviolence in relation to internalized, traumatic violence?

Yoder's work provides a good starting place for addressing these questions. Although Yoder does not explicitly attend to internalized violence, his writings contain resources that shed light on how faith communities can participate in the transformation of this dimension of violence. Specifically, his reading of the narratives of Jesus opens up the possibility that although we may become sites of violence through social construction, this does not express the totality of our being. Individuals and communities also can be formed in ways that transform internal violence and integrate nonviolence into their identities, so that they become not only sites of violence but also sites of grace.

In the pages ahead, I explore how Christian communities may foster (or impede) the healing of internalized, traumatic violence and the integration of nonviolence. Before turning to this task, however, I first want to consider the dynamics of internalized violence: how this violence can become integrated into our identities and the ongoing effects of this harm. I thus turn in the next chapter to trauma studies, an interdisciplinary field that analyzes trauma as a destructive form of violence that can become deeply embedded within individuals and communities as they are formed in history over time.

NOTES

1. See Richard J. Mouw, "Foreword," in *The Royal Priesthood: Essays Ecclesiological and Ecumenical*, ed. Michael G. Cartwright (Grand Rapids, MI: Eerdmans, 1994), vii–ix.

2. Mark Thiessen Nation, "John H. Yoder, Ecumenical Neo-Anabaptist: A Biographical Sketch," in *The Wisdom of the Cross*, eds. Stanley Hauerwas, et al. (Grand Rapids, MI: Eerdmans, 1999), 1.

3. See Yoder, *The Priestly Kingdom* (Notre Dame, IN: University of Notre Dame Press, 1984), 4.

4. Yoder, "How H. Richard Niebuhr Reasoned: A Critique of *Christ and Culture*," in *Authentic Transformation: A New Vision of Christ and Culture*, eds. Glen H. Stassen, D. M. Yeager, and John Howard Yoder (Nashville, KY: Abingdon Press, 1996), 73.

5. Yoder, *The Politics of Jesus* (Grand Rapids, MI: Eerdmans, 1994), 95.
6. Yoder, *The Politics of Jesus*, 95.
7. Reinhard Hütter, "The Church: Midwife of History or Witness of the Eschaton?" *Journal of Religious Ethics* 18 (Spring 1990): 40.
8. "The Original Revolution," in *The Original Revolution: Essays on Christian Pacifism* (Scottdale, PA: Herald Press, 1971; reprinting by Wipf and Stock Publishers, Eugene, OR: 1998), 29.
9. "The Original Revolution," 19.
10. "The Original Revolution," 28.
11. See Yoder, *The Politics of Jesus.*, ch. 2.
12. Yoder, *The Politics of Jesus*, ch.2. Yoder conflates the accounts in Luke and John here.
13. Yoder, "The Biblical Mandate for Evangelical Social Action," in *For the Nations: Essays Public and Evangelical* (Grand Rapids, MI: Eerdmans, 1997), 191.
14. Yoder, *The Politics of Jesus*, 36.
15. David Toole, *Waiting for Godot in Sarajevo* (Boulder, CO: Westview Press, 1998), 214.
16. Yoder, *Body Politics*, 81n5.
17. Yoder, *Body Politics*, 81n5.
18. Yoder, *Body Politics*, ix.
19. Yoder, *The Politics of Jesus*, 229–30.
20. Yoder, "The Believers Church and the Arms Race," in *For the Nations: Essays Public and Evangelical* (Grand Rapids, MI: Eerdmans, 1997), 150–51.
21. Yoder, *The Politics of Jesus*, 232.
22. Yoder, *The Politics of Jesus*, 137.
23. Yoder, *The Politics of Jesus*, 137–38.
24. Yoder, *The Politics of Jesus*, 141.
25. Yoder, *The Politics of Jesus*, 141.
26. Yoder, *The Politics of Jesus*, 142.
27. Yoder, *The Politics of Jesus*, 144–45.
28. Berkhof, *Christ and the Powers*, translated by John Howard Yoder (Scottdale, PA: Herald Press, 1977). qtd. in Yoder, *The Politics of Jesus*, 146.
29. Yoder, *The Politics of Jesus*, 145. Yoder distinguishes between "subordination," "subjection," and "submission." He claims that the term subjection "carries a connotation of being thrown down and run over . . . *submission* . . . [has the] connotation of passivity. Sub*ordi*nation means the acceptance of an *order*, as it exists, but with the new meaning given to it by the fact that one's acceptance of it is willing and meaningfully motivated" (*The Politics of Jesus*, 172). Although this may seem to suggest that Christians should adopt a quietistic attitude toward the current social order, Yoder argues that this is not the case. He makes a further distinction between "subordination" and "obedience." For Yoder, the "conscientious objector who refuses to do what the government demands, but still remains under the sovereignty of that government and accepts the penalties which it imposes, or the Christian who refuses to worship Caesar but still permits Caesar to put him or her to death, is being subordinate even though not obeying" (*The Politics of Jesus*, 209). The church that adopts a stance of subordination should, therefore, still work toward social change by identifying and seeking to remove through nonviolent

means "one abuse at a time" ("The Racial Revolution in Theological Perspective," in *For the Nations,* 119). In so doing, it resists injustice in ways that break the cycles of violence already set in motion.

30. Berkhof, *Christ and the Powers,* qtd. in Yoder, *The Politics of Jesus,* 146.

31. Berkhof, *Christ and the Powers,* qtd. in Yoder, *The Politics of Jesus,* 146.

32. Yoder, *The Politics of Jesus,* 160.

33. Yoder, *What Would You Do? A Serious Answer to a Standard Question* (Scottdale, PA: Herald Press, Inc., 1992), 35.

34. Berkhof, *Christ and the Powers,* qtd. in Yoder, *The Politics of Jesus,* 147.

35. Yoder, *The Politics of Jesus,* 150.

36. Yoder, "The Believers Church and the Arms Race," in *For the Nations,* 153.

37. Yoder, *Body Politics: Five Practices of the Christian Community before the Watching World* (Nashville, TN: Discipleship Resources, 1992), 78.

38. "The Otherness of the Church," 62.

39. Yoder, "How H. Richard Niebuhr Reasoned: A Critique of *Christ and Culture,* 70.

40. "The Otherness of the Church," in *The Royal Priesthood,* 56.

41. "Why Ecclesiology is Social Ethics," in *The Royal Priesthood,* 108–9.

42. "A People in the World," in *The Royal Priesthood,* 80.

43. Yoder, *The Politics of Jesus,* 158.

44. Nancey Murphy, "John Howard Yoder's Systematic Defense of Christian Pacifism," in *The Wisdom of the Cross: Essays in Honor of John Howard Yoder,* eds. Stanley Hauerwas et al. (Grand Rapids, MI: Wm. B. Eerdmans, 1999), 65.

45. Nancey Murphy," John Howard Yoder's Systematic Defense of Christian Pacifism," 60.

46. Yoder states that Niebuhr made an important contribution to theology in "making real the omnipresence of sin, even when mixed with the best of intentions." "Reinhold Niebuhr and Christian Pacifism," *Mennonite Quarterly Review* 29 (April 1955): 117.

47. Craig Carter, *The Politics of the Cross: The Theology and Social Ethics of John Howard Yoder* (Grand Rapids, MI: Brazos Press, 2001), 148.

48. See Yoder's introduction to *The Priestly Kingdom* (Notre Dame, IN: Notre Dame University Press, 1984), 5.

49. Yoder, "How H. Richard Niebuhr Reasoned," 77.

50. "A People in the World," 74.

51. "A People in the World," 75.

52. "A People in the World," 75.

53. "A People in the World," 75.

54. "A People in the World," 74–75.

55. "The Otherness of the Church," 56.

56. Yoder, "Christ the Hope of the World," in *The Original Revolution,* 180.

57. Yoder asserts that in the writings of Paul and John, the world "is pretty clearly being thought of as a coherent unity, polarized over against the new world of the gospel, the message of the new age. But there are times and places where that simplicity doesn't fit and we can't reason that clearly . . . We can't simply say 'yes' or 'no,' the world is out there and we are over here. There are good reasons for that. Complexity is not all the work of the devil. Partly it is the progress of the gospel" ("The Believers Church and the Arms Race," *For the Nations,* 151).

58. Yoder, "The Believers Church and the Arms Race," 151–52.
59. Yoder, "The Believers Church and the Arms Race," 150.
60. Yoder, "The Believers Church and the Arms Race," 151.
61. Yoder, "The Believers Church and the Arms Race," 152.
62. Stanley Hauerwas makes this point about Yoder's interpretation of the world in *The Peacable Kingdom* (Notre Dame, IN: The University of Notre Dame Press, 1983), 101.
63. Yoder, "The Otherness of the Church," 56.
64. Yoder, "The Believers Church and the Arms Race," 157.
65. Yoder, "The Believers Church and the Arms Race," 157.
66. Yoder, "The Believers Church and the Arms Race," 156.
67. Yoder, "A People in the World," 78.
68. Yoder, "The Paradigmatic Public Role of God's People," in *For the Nations*, 27–28.
69. Toole, *Waiting for Godot in Sarajevo*, 224.
70. Yoder, "The Biblical Mandate for Evangelical Social Action," in *For the Nations*, 185.
71. Yoder, "The Biblical Mandate for Evangelical Social Action," 185.
72. Yoder, *The Christian Witness to the State* (Newtown, KS: Faith and Life Press, 1964), 20–21.
73. Yoder, *The Christian Witness to the State*, 20.
74. Yoder, *The Christian Witness to the State*, 19.
75. Yoder, *The Christian Witness to the State*, 21.
76. Yoder, *The Christian Witness to the State*, 21.
77. Yoder, *The Christian Witness to the State*, 39.
78. Yoder, *The Christian Witness to the State*, 41. While Yoder speaks of middle axioms early in his career, he later abandons the use of the term. See J. Denny Weaver, "The Yoder Legacy: Whither the Second Generation?" *The Mennonite Quarterly Review* 77, no. 3 (July 2003): 469–70.
79. Yoder, "The Biblical Mandate for Evangelical Social Action," 182.
80. Yoder, "The Racial Revolution in Theological Perspective," in *For the Nations*, 111.
81. Yoder understands this suffering to be the price of one's social nonconformity, not all experiences of suffering. *The Politics of Jesus*, 129.
82. Yoder, "The Biblical Mandate for Evangelical Social Action," 182.
83. J. Denny Weaver," "Theology in the Mirror of the Martyred and Oppressed," in *The Wisdom of the Cross*, 424.
84. Lisa Adler and L. H. M. Ling use the terms "internal" and "external" violence in their article "From Practice to Theory: Toward a Dissident-Feminist Reconstruction of Nonviolence," *Gandhi Marg* 16 (January–March 1995): 462–480.
85. For a critique of traditional views of nonviolence that assume an understanding of violence as "external," see Lisa Adler and L. H. M. Ling, "From Practice to Theory."
86. For example, see Judith Lewis Herman, *Trauma and Recovery* (New York: Basicbooks, 1992), and Bessel van der Kolk, Lars Weisaeth, and Onno van der Hart, *Traumatic Stress: The Effects of Overwhelming Experience on Mind, Body, and Society* (New York: The Guilford Press), 1996.
87. See Adler and Ling, "From Practice to Theory," 467–68.

88. For a summary of different understandings of social construction, see Serene Jones, *Cartographies of Grace: Feminist Theory and Theology* (Minneapolis: Fortress Press, 2000), 31–42.

89. King, *Why We Can't Wait* (New York: Signet Classic, 2000), 69.

90. King, *Why We Can't Wait,* 70.

91. King, "The Current Crisis in Race Relations," in *A Testament of Hope: The Essential Writings of Martin Luther* King, Jr., ed. James Melvin Washington (San Francisco: Harper & Row, 1986), 87.

92. Judith Lewis Herman, *Trauma and Recovery* (New York: Basic Books, 1992), 113.

93. See Ian Angus and Sut Jhally, qtd. in bell hooks, "Liberation Scenes," *Yearning: Race, Gender, and Cultural Politics* (Boston: South End Press, 1993), 5.

94. See hooks, "Liberation Scenes."

95. Russell, *The Church with AIDS: Renewal in the Midst of Crisis,* ed. Letty M. Russell (Louisville, KY: Westminster John Knox Press, 1990), 26.

2

Trauma and the Fragmentation of the Self

In her book *Too Scared to Cry*, psychiatrist Lenore Terr tells the story of a group of children who were kidnapped while riding their school bus home from a summer program in Chowchilla, California. As she describes it, the kidnapping began when a masked gunman and his companion stopped their bus and took charge, forcing the children out of the vehicle and into two different vans. After hours of confinement with no food or light, the children were ordered by their captors to get off the vans and climb into a hole in the ground, from which they eventually escaped. While they were declared in good condition by doctors who examined them immediately after the ordeal, those who knew them well soon came to realize that something was wrong. The children—and some of their siblings and friends who were not present during the kidnapping—suffered from nightmares, feelings of helplessness, fear of death, anxiety, and a sense of pessimism about their personal futures. They experienced the kidnapping not merely as an event in the past, but as a present reality that shaped their lives in many ways.[1]

This story of the Chowchilla children captures well the essence of "trauma" or "traumatic violence," violence that leads to patterns of psychic wounding. In recent years, scholars and clinicians have analyzed trauma as a particularly acute form of harm that can become internal to the self over time. They have observed that some trauma survivors, like the kidnapped children, remain unable psychologically to "let go" of their traumatic experiences. Instead, the memories and emotions associated with these events remain powerful and become deeply entrenched within their bodies, minds, and souls. In this way, trauma survivors become sites of violence:

They hold within them the reality of the violence they have experienced as ever present, even as they move through time.

In this chapter I draw on the interdisciplinary field of contemporary "trauma studies" or "trauma theory" to analyze this form of internal violence and its implications for Christian nonviolence. After a brief discussion of the origins of trauma studies, I examine what constitutes a "trauma" or "traumatic event" and its long-term effects, both those included in the well-known clinical description of post-traumatic stress disorder (PTSD) and those not discussed under this category. In exploring the dynamics of trauma, I focus on how it can fragment the self as it moves from the outside in, disrupting the survivor's ability to integrate memories, create a coherent personal narrative, establish healthy interpersonal relationships, and construct a positive vision for his or her future.

In presenting a picture of the traumatized self as deeply fractured or fragmented, contemporary trauma studies requires us to rethink traditional Christian understandings of nonviolence. Rather than focusing only on external violence, we must consider as well how faith communities can resist and transform the ongoing effects of internalized, traumatic violence that many of their members experience. While not all trauma survivors who participate in religious communities benefit from them, some do, and trauma studies gives us a language and conceptuality for understanding how. It offers a detailed description of the ways in which trauma affects people psychologically, spiritually, and physically; furthermore, it explores (as I will discuss in chapter 3) how traumatized persons can work to transform the effects of trauma through healing. In these ways, trauma studies illuminates an often-overlooked dimension of nonviolence: the creation of communal contexts in which traumatized persons can survive and flourish.

TRAUMA AND TRAUMATIC STRESS

Trauma studies is an odd academic discipline. Unlike most other disciplines, it is comprised of clinicians and scholars from different fields who all study trauma and, therefore, contribute to what many in the humanities now call "trauma theory."[2] Although there are differing accounts of the origins of this field, those who study trauma ("trauma scholars" or "trauma theorists") generally agree that the modern analysis of trauma began in the late 1800s. At this time the British physician John Erichsen noted the stress symptoms suffered by railway accident victims and described these symptoms as the result of an injury to the spine.[3] Near the turn of the century, the term "trauma" acquired more psychological meaning when figures such as Sigmund Freud, Pierre Janet, and Alfred Binet began to study the injury to the mind that resulted from sudden emotional shock.[4] One example that captured their interest was the "hysteria" found in some females, which Freud initially attributed to their unconscious, repressed memories of sexual violence (a theory he later denied).[5] The study of trauma subsequently tapered off in the early 1900s but resurfaced after World War I when veterans exhibited signs of what people later called "shell shock"—a topic that commanded significant medical and public attention again during World War II. While interest in trauma declined again after World War II, it reemerged in public consciousness when psychiatrists, social workers, and activists began to discuss the psychological effects of the Viet Nam War on its veterans.[6]

Since the years following the Viet Nam War, the study of trauma has expanded to incorporate a broader range of questions and concerns. In the 1970s and 1980s women's advocates began examining the psychological effects of sexual abuse on women and children, extending the discussion of trauma beyond the problem of war neuroses and accidents.[7] Recently, the conversation has moved into the field of psychobiology, where scholars study how trauma affects the brain and multiple levels of biological functioning.[8] In the field of literature, writers working on Holocaust literature broach the subject of trauma in a different way: They ask how we can write about events that are so horrible it seems we cannot even describe them in words.[9] Many legal and political theorists interested in trauma consider how collective violence harms whole communities and countries, such as in the case of South Africa or Rwanda—and what healing involves for a nation shattered by this violence.[10] And some scholars who work in the fields of history and cultural studies analyze trauma by examining topics such as the Middle Passage and racial subjugation during slavery in North America and its aftermath.[11]

While these trauma theorists approach the study of trauma from different perspectives, they share the goal of understanding the dynamics of violence that leads to patterns of psychic wounding. Using a variety of methodologies, they analyze how trauma affects individuals and communities, both in the immediate aftermath of the violence and in the long-term. In undertaking this task, they often begin with an account of what constitutes a "trauma"—a term whose meaning has evolved over the years.

As poststructuralist literary critic Cathy Caruth observes, the term trauma (in English and German) derives from the Greek *trauma*, or wound, which originally referred to a blow inflicted on the body.[12] In later years, especially in the psychiatric and medical fields, "trauma" came to denote events that inflicted wounds not only on the body but also on the mind.[13] More recently, scholars in the social sciences have developed this latter understanding of trauma by defining it more precisely as an extremely stressful event that elicits an intense sense of helplessness, fear, and loss of control.[14] With this definition, they indicate that trauma differs from "normal," everyday stresses, such as a bad day at work or a high-pressure examination at school. Such experiences can certainly produce anxiety, but they do not render us utterly overwhelmed and terrified. Trauma generates stress of a different magnitude—stress that is particularly intense and can have effects that last for months, years, or even decades after the trauma has ended.

When describing what constitutes a trauma, trauma scholars often distinguish between the terms "trauma" and "traumatic stress" or "post-traumatic stress disorder" (PTSD).[15] Whereas trauma refers simply to an extremely stressful event or experience, "traumatic stress" or "post-traumatic stress disorder" represents an interrelated cluster of symptoms that can develop in its aftermath. Neurobiologists Alexander McFarlane and Bessel van der Kolk broadly describe traumatic stress as "the result of a failure of time to heal all wounds."[16] For those who develop PTSD—for those who are traumatized—the trauma is not simply in the past. It is constantly re-experienced through repetitive phenomena such as nightmares, flashbacks, and intrusive memories of the trauma.

In describing how PTSD develops, trauma theorists note that it is normal for those victims who have experienced a trauma to become preoccupied with it, experiencing involuntary, intrusive thoughts about the trauma that are accompanied by painful emotions.[17] In many cases, this preoccupation allows the survivor to cognitively and emotionally come to terms with the event and to incorporate it into their personal narrative as a difficult experience in the past. For some victims, however, this preoccupation with the trauma does not lessen over time. Instead of gradually remembering the event less frequently and experiencing the emotions it evokes less intensely, they continue to think of the trauma often and experience every memory of it as if this trauma were happening again. This repeated reliving of the trauma increases the victim's level of distress, often interfering with their ability to perform the tasks of their daily lives.[18] Re-experiencing the trauma leads some survivors to develop an interrelated cluster of biological, emotional, psychological, and cognitive symptoms that trauma theorists now associate with PTSD.[19]

Trauma theorists contend that the development of PTSD begins with the experience of an event in history and not with an incident that was merely imagined or misinterpreted.[20] At the same time, however, the survivor's subjective interpretation plays a role in determining if an event is traumatic.[21] Whether or not victims become traumatized depends not only on the nature of the event but also on their response to it—how threatened and helpless they feel during the event—and on the meaning they attach to it in its aftermath. Given this subjectivity, trauma theorists observe that we cannot easily determine why some survivors develop PTSD while others do not. Two people can experience the same event and respond to it quite differently.[22] Certain factors, however, place some persons at greater risk for traumatization than others. One can group these factors, which do not alone explain the onset of PTSD, into four categories.[23]

First, the kind of the trauma can help to determine how the victim responds.[24] Interpersonal traumas or traumas of human origin, such as physical abuse, often produce greater degrees of traumatization than "natural" or impersonal traumas such as earthquakes, hurricanes, and floods. The former are more likely to fragment human relationships and to diminish the survivor's sense of self-worth.[25] In addition, they are more often repeated over time and thus have cumulative effects.[26] For example, in situations of incest and domestic violence, the repetitive nature of the traumas can lead to a deeper fragmentation of the survivor's (and perpetrator's) self.

Second, factors related to the individual trauma victim can increase his or her chance of developing PTSD. For example, the victim's genetic vulnerability to being overwhelmed and certain personality traits, such as neuroticism and introversion, can make the onset of traumatization more likely.[27] The survivor's age and developmental phase can further influence the post-traumatic response pattern; some scholars theorize that since one's psychological coping mechanisms develop over time, young children are particularly at risk for post-traumatic stress disorder.[28] Prior traumatization and the victim's response during the trauma also can contribute to the development of PTSD. If the victim has experienced other traumas, and if he or she panics or goes numb during the event, traumatization will more likely result.

An additional factor related to the individual trauma victim is whether he or she has received advance preparation for how to handle the trauma. According to Arieh Shalev, adequate training can limit the effects of stress by reducing victims' uncertainty in the face of trauma. It also can increase their sense of control during the event and give them skills that enable them to act effectively in the midst of the crisis.[29] For example, medical personnel trained to handle emergency situations are less vulnerable to traumatization when they see a serious accident than witnesses who have no such training. Those who have not prepared for such an event will more likely "freeze" or surrender, which increases their chance of experiencing prolonged distress.[30]

Third, the cultural context surrounding the individual survivor can shape their response, making it either more or less likely that traumatization will develop. Trauma theorists assert that cultures can help survivors cope by creating systems of meaning or belief that provide them with ways to process their loss and regain a sense of hope in the midst of despair. For instance, many cultures have specific customs and rituals designed to help people express and deal with their grief.[31] Such cultural performances can mitigate the survivor's pain and reduce their risk of developing traumatic stress.

The strength of the survivor's social support network is a fourth factor that helps determine whether a trauma leads to traumatization. While support from family, friends, or others does not necessarily prevent traumatic stress, it lessens the chance that it will develop by giving survivors psychological, emotional, and financial resources that can help them to cope.[32] Unfortunately, such support often remains unavailable, especially for those who experience forms of violence that society deems taboo, such as sexual assault.[33] While after a collective trauma such as 9/11 or Hurricane Katrina people rush to help victims, they often respond to survivors of individual traumas with judgment and blame. For traumatized people, this response can be debilitating. When others discount their stories, blame them for their misfortunes, or treat them as though they bear a stigma, survivors relive the isolation they experienced during their traumas. This again cuts them off from the support system that could help restore their sense of safety and stability.[34]

McFarlane and van der Kolk argue that just as individuals often do not offer support to trauma survivors, some institutions, such as insurance companies and the armed forces, deny the prevalence of trauma and the extent of its impact.[35] This denial may stem from financial motivations, such as when insurance companies seek to avoid paying damage claims to survivors.[36] In other instances, institutions minimize the effects of trauma to enhance the credibility of their own views or actions. For example, political and military forces that wage war generally remain reluctant to acknowledge the trauma they cause others to endure, since recognizing this harm may undermine public support.

At times, the medical field has also undermined the availability of social support by helping to foster a culture of denial. Although psychiatrists have studied trauma since the nineteenth century, the American Psychiatric Association's *Diagnostic Statistical Manual of Mental Disorders* did not include PTSD until 1980.[37] Even then, the manual minimized trauma's prevalence by defining traumatic events as "outside the range of ordinary human experiences."[38] Research studies call this definition into question. They estimate that in the United States, approximately 20–33 percent of girls and 6–9 percent of boys are sexually abused by age eighteen.[39] They further indicate that one of every three women in the United States will experience sexual assault.[40] In addition, millions of people endure traumas such as war and natural disasters. As Judith Herman observes, trauma "must be considered a common part of human experience; only the fortunate find it unusual. Traumatic events are extraordinary, not because they occur rarely, but rather because they overwhelm the ordinary human adaptations to life."[41]

FEMINIST RESPONSES TO CLINICAL THEORIES OF TRAUMA

The description of trauma and traumatization that I have offered so far draws on "clinical" or "medicalized" paradigms for studying trauma, which some call "traditional" or "clinical" trauma theory. Clinical trauma theory seeks to understand the ongoing effects of trauma on individuals. To this end, its proponents generate a list of symptoms (which I discuss below) that often result from traumatic violence. While this list contributes much to our understanding of trauma, several feminist scholars have criticized this approach. These scholars share the conviction that traditional paradigms for studying trauma have a significant flaw: They focus too much on the individual victim and not enough on the social and political contexts in which trauma takes place.

Some feminists who study trauma contend that traditional decontextualizing approaches to trauma studies obscure the ways in which social inequalities create conditions that sanction traumatic violence and compound its effects.[42] Systems of oppression, such as poverty and racism, place some people at greater risk for experiencing trauma than others. For example, women of color who work in the homes of white men and their families historically have been particularly vulnerable to sexual abuse.[43] In addition to increasing the risk of trauma, social injustice makes it harder for some people to resist or recover from their traumas by restricting their access to social and material resources.[44] A poor woman who endures domestic violence, for instance, lacks the financial resources that may help her to resist and break free from the violence. The violence in her home adds to the stress her poverty has already induced, and she lives without the means to address the difficulties that stem from both forms of harm.

Feminist scholars assert that decontextualizing approaches to trauma studies lead us to unfairly blame and stigmatize trauma survivors.[45] We tend to ask "what's wrong" with the individual victim, rather than what's wrong with our society that subjects people to so many kinds of violent harm. Often, those who encounter trauma survivors account for their symptoms by pointing to perceived deficiencies in their character, such as an inability to cope with stressful situations or an inherent pathology. However, focusing only on factors related to the individual obscures the fact that their symptoms are a normal response to violence and that this response stems partly from their experiences of injustice.

Feminists who criticize clinical trauma theory thus propose an alternative approach. They begin by noting that the real problem is not the victim but the offenders and the contexts in which traumas take place.[46] To bring the social dimensions of trauma into focus, they expand the definition of trauma in two ways. First, they speak of "insidious traumas," forms of harm that are not overtly physically violent but that nonetheless "do violence to a person's soul or spirit."[47] Within this category, they include experiences of institutional abuse that produce extreme levels of stress, such as confinement in prisons or concentration camps. They also include chronic experiences of oppression that devalue people. For example, some scholars claim that racism and sexism can constitute chronic trauma that produces symptoms similar to those suffered by victims of overt physical violence: anxiety, depression, loss of voice, low self-esteem, and hypersensitivity to the threat of danger.[48] note, however, that feminists who study trauma do not simply equate the terms "trauma" and "oppression." Some experiences of oppression are not traumatic, and not all people who experience oppression are traumatized. In developing the notion of insidious traumas, then, these scholars do not mean to say that all oppressed people have post-traumatic stress in the clinical sense. Rather, they are suggesting that clinical theories generally fail to sufficiently address both the breadth of experiences that can produce traumalike symptoms and the ways in which experiences of oppression may compound the long-term effects of traumatic violence.

Second, some feminist clinicians and scholars who emphasize the social dimensions of trauma expand its definition by speaking of "indirect" or "secondary" traumas. According to Maria Root, indirect traumas involve being traumatized by the harms that another person sustains. This can happen when one witnesses a trauma—as, for example, when one sees dead bodies removed from an accident scene or a parent beaten or killed. It can also happen when one listens to the stories of others who have been victimized—as do therapists who work with trauma survivors.[49] Some children of Holocaust survivors manifest another form of indirect trauma when they exhibit trauma symptoms, even though they did not experience firsthand the horrors their parents faced.[50] In these instances, the trauma stories that the children hear from their parents become part of their life story as well, an integral part of their own identities.

Laura Brown identifies still another kind of indirect trauma when she states that trauma symptoms can spread laterally within oppressed social groups as well as intergenerationally.[51] As examples, she mentions gays and lesbians who fear being assaulted for their choice in partners. She also cites the experiences of people of color in the United States, who contend with racially motivated violence and discrimination. In addition, Brown observes that most North American women know that they are always vulnerable to sexual violation. As a result, even if they have not been directly victimized and do not have posttraumatic stress dissorder, they may show symptoms similar to those of rape victims though to a lesser degree. For example, they may experience intense fear when alone at night or go numb in response to advances from men. Brown concludes that such insidious traumas should make us question our society in which so many people confront traumatic stressors on a daily basis.[52]

While feminists broaden traditional trauma studies beyond its focus on the individual victim, they do not want to ignore the specific effects that trauma has on survivors. Like those who work within a clinical paradigm, feminist trauma scholars strive to understand the ways in which traumatic violence can fragment the self over time. They, too, see trauma as an invasive reality and recognize that those who experience it suffer profound harm, not only by the trauma itself but even more by the symptoms that develop in its aftermath. What, specifically, are these symptoms, the long-term effects of trauma that can break down or fragment the self? To address this question requires exploring how trauma theorists describe the common features of traumatic stress, including those that appear in the clinical description of PTSD and those that do not.

COMMON FEATURES OF TRAUMATIZATION

While it is impossible to universalize the effects of trauma on individuals, trauma theorists find that survivors of diverse forms of trauma sometimes exhibit similar physical, psychological, and behavioral responses.[53] Given this commonality, they often speak in generalized terms about the effects of trauma. This does not mean, of course, that all traumatized persons manifest every symptom described and to the same degree. Coping with combat, for example, does not raise precisely the same issues as coping with an accident.[54] But given that in the midst of the differences among survivors' experiences and responses there exist similarities as well, trauma scholars indicate that it is justified to describe common patterns of response that often persist in trauma's aftermath.

INTRUSIVE MEMORIES AND HYPERAROUSAL

Trauma theorists contend that some survivors become preoccupied with their traumas in the aftermath of these events and experience intrusive memories about them that they cannot control. At times, these intrusive memories take the form of flashbacks in which the survivor mentally "views" the trauma as they would a movie scene: They are immersed in the memory of it and can visualize it vividly in their minds as if it were happening again.[55] Other survivors may not actually "see" their trauma in this way but instead re-experience an image, smell, or sensation in their body that they had at the time of the trauma. For example, a man who was physically attacked may have the same pain in his arm that he felt when his attacker grabbed it. Those trauma survivors who cannot consciously remember their traumas may not have any idea why they are having these sensations. But they may experience them as quite distressing nonetheless.

While some survivors find that this replaying of painful memories enables them to modify the emotions associated with the trauma and to integrate this event into their life story, others remain unable to adapt to the trauma and become overwhelmed.[56] Instead of gradually fading, their memories of the trauma persist and become increasingly painful. Each time they remember the event they experience it as if it were occurring again in the present. For some survivors, these intrusive memories lead to hyperarousal, a condition in which people experience extreme physiological and psychological arousal in response to certain stimuli in their environment.[57] Judith Herman notes that for those who develop this extreme sensitivity, even small reminders can evoke memories of the trauma, "which often return with all the vividness and emotional force of the original event."[58]

At a most basic level, hyperarousal is thus a condition in which a person loses the ability to regulate arousal and how he or she responds to stress. It is like having one's "fight or flight" system turn on too easily and too often. On its own, the fight or flight response signals potentially dangerous situations and helps people to manage them. As van der Kolk observes, ordinarily during stressful events victims experience an adrenaline rush that enables them to assess the situation accurately and to respond quickly. However, the chronic hyperarousal that some traumatized people experience diminishes the effectiveness of their stress response and distorts their ability to assess incoming stimuli. Constantly on the alert for the return of their trauma, they may be unable to accurately process information about their internal states as well as external cues. As a result, they may have difficulty telling when they are imperiled and panic easily, which can cause them either to freeze or to overreact.[59]

Some trauma theorists maintain that experiencing even a single trauma can cause changes in brain chemistry that make survivors more sensitive to adrenaline rushes for years after the trauma.[60] However, hyperarousal becomes more entrenched when the abuse is chronic, such as in many cases of child sexual abuse. Repeated abuse disrupts the normal patterns of bodily functions, such as eating and sleeping.[61] As a result, chronically traumatized persons often suffer from hypervigilance, exaggerated startle response, restlessness, and difficulty sleeping and concentrating (all symptoms of hyperarousal).[62] Given their inability to discriminate between neutral environmental stimuli and genuine indicators of danger, those who experience hyperarousal tend to perceive the world—both the external world and their internal world—as unsafe.[63] As Ronnie Janoff-Bulman notes, this leads them to feel "a double dose of anxiety." One stems from the realization of their own vulnerability, and the other from the challenge that the trauma poses to their conceptual systems: "The very assumptions that had provided psychological coherence and stability in a complex world are . . . shattered."[64]

RESPONSES TO HYPERAROUSAL: AVOIDANCE AND NUMBING

To cope with their hyperarousal, traumatized persons often enter into a state of emotional numbness. Overwhelmed by the painful feelings that intrusive memories evoke, they gradually withdraw from emotions and physical sensations. According to van der Kolk and McFarlane, trauma survivors may not consciously detach emotionally. Instead, this response may happen because hyperarousal drains the biological and psychological resources needed to experience a variety of emotions.[65] When traumatized people do not automatically experience this dampening of affect, they sometimes use drugs or alcohol to numb their pain and make them feel "dead to the world."[66]

For some survivors, emotional withdrawal does not simply replace the hyperarousal that can develop after a trauma. Instead, both states alternately persist. The victim oscillates between experiencing intense, painful emotions and feeling nothing at all.[67] While some trauma theorists believe that this dialectic prohibits recovery, others argue that it can have significant adaptive value. For example, Janoff-Bulman suggests that survivors who exhibit both responses are moving back and forth between the need to confront their traumas (intrusive recollections) and the desire to protect themselves from their painful memories (numbing).[68] This combination of intrusive recollections and numbing can facilitate recovery by enabling survivors to come to terms with their traumatic experiences. It can give them a chance to process their traumatic memories without becoming overwhelmed by the intense emotions they evoke.[69]

In addition to experiencing a generalized numbness, some traumatized persons respond to hyperarousal by (consciously or unconsciously) avoiding specific triggers that remind them of their traumas. Eve Carlson and her colleagues identify three types of avoidance: emotional (which can take the form of numbing to escape the pain of distressing emotions); cognitive ("spacing out" when facing cues associated with traumatic experiences); and behavioral (staying away from people or situations that may remind the survivors of their traumas).[70] A war veteran may experience dampened affect that is a form of emotional avoidance. Similarly, a sexual abuse survivor may demonstrate cognitive dissociation by spacing out when witnessing media coverage of sexual violence. And a car accident victim may exhibit behavioral avoidance by refusing to return to the site of the crash. In steering clear of this site, the victim can avoid remembering the trauma and experiencing the painful emotions this memory would evoke.[71]

DISSOCIATION AND TRAUMATIC MEMORY

One form of emotional numbing is dissociation, a splitting of the mind that can occur during a stressful event and in subsequent periods of stress.[72] In dissociation, aspects of the trauma—such as thoughts, actions, emotions, or sensations—are separated from the victim's conscious awareness. As Sandra Bloom observes, most of the time people know what they just did and what is going on around them. Sometimes, however, this is not the case. For example, some people occasionally get in their cars and begin to drive, only to discover that when they arrive at their destination they cannot remember anything about the journey.[73] This capacity to mentally "go away" for a period of time can become a defense mechanism in situations of trauma. When people mentally dissociate, they detach psychologically and emotionally so that they do not really experience what is happening to them. In a mild form of dissociation, they may feel a sense of unreality. In more extreme instances, survivors sometimes mentally leave their bodies and watch the trauma from a distance, as if it were happening to someone else.[74]

As a defense mechanism, dissociation serves the purpose of protecting victims from confronting the full emotional and cognitive impact of their traumas. For some survivors, it prevents them from becoming overwhelmed by keeping parts of the traumatic experiences concealed and outside of conscious awareness.[75] In addition to blocking out conscious memories of the trauma, dissociation can protect victims by inducing a state of emotional numbness. However, trauma theorists emphasize that dissociation does not always achieve this numbness. Sometimes, survivors who dissociate experience painful feelings such as fear, despair, confusion, and aloneness. In such cases, they may feel the full emotional intensity of the traumas without knowing the historical cause. For instance, they may have anxiety without understanding why.[76]

Some trauma theorists explain dissociation by studying how memory and traumatic memory work. Although researchers do not entirely agree on this issue, a number of scholars believe that the human brain contains two main memory systems.[77] One is a language-based system that consists of conscious awareness of facts or events ("declarative" or "explicit" memory). According to Bloom, this system verbally encodes all our new experiences, filing them away in a "knowledge base" that we acquire from birth onward. The other memory system, which does not require words or thoughts, contains unconscious memories of skills, habits, reflexive actions, and emotional responses ("nondeclarative," "implicit," or "procedural" memory).[78] Bloom asserts that this system attaches emotional meaning to our experiences, "even before we recognize what we are reacting to or what we are feeling."[79] Usually, these two memory systems work in parallel and in a coordinated way, enabling us to perform complex tasks such as driving a car while processing directions about where we are going.[80] As we engage in such tasks, we can be consciously aware of information contained in the declarative memory system while simultaneously drawing on our procedural memory.[81]

Under extremely stressful conditions, however, the declarative memory system may fail. When this occurs, people lose the capacity to translate their experiences into verbal categories, and their minds switch to a way of thinking dominated by physical sensations and emotions.[82] Some trauma scholars believe this is what happens when individuals dissociate: Traumatic memories are separated from ordinary consciousness and not integrated into a personal narrative. They are stored as sensory perceptions, rather than in verbal-linguistic categories.[83] When traumatic memories are organized on a nonverbal level, they recur as nightmares, flashbacks, bodily sensations, or behavioral reenactments of the trauma.[84] Thus, after some traumas a dynamic of mimetic replay is set in motion in which traumatic memories continue to circulate in the victim's psychic and physical structures but remain unattached to those memories that constitute their personal narrative or life story. For survivors, this recirculation of the traumatic memories has a gripping or totalizing force. It comes to dominate their life, making them feel stuck in the past, disconnected from the present, and unable to anticipate the future with hope.[85]

While some trauma survivors dissociate during a trauma, others do not. Many can remember and describe the trauma in its immediate aftermath, although it may take a while to process it emotionally.[86] In general, victims are more likely to dissociate when they are young and when their traumas are repeated. Some trauma theorists also note that social contexts can influence how the victim remembers the event. In a study comparing the traumatic memories of Holocaust survivors to those of child abuse victims, Laurence Kirmayer finds that the social conditions or "landscapes" in which survivors remember and recount their traumas make the latter group more susceptible to dissociation. Child abuse victims are more likely than Holocaust survivors to dissociate, partly because society does not widely recognize personal abuse stories as human catastrophes.[87] Instead, it often denies that such abuse even happens. In Kirmayer's view,

> The difference is between a public space of solidarity and a private space of shame. Trauma shared by a whole community creates a potential public space for retelling. If a community agrees traumatic events occurred and weaves this fact into its identity, then collective memory survives and individual memory can find a place (albeit transformed) within that landscape. If a family or a community agrees that a trauma did not happen, then it vanishes from collective memory and the possibility for individual memory is severely strained.[88]

Kirmayer's analysis indicates that the individual's remembering and forgetting are deeply shaped by the public's response to their trauma. When the public acknowledges the trauma and offers compassion, dissociation will less likely occur.

Even when dissociation does happen, the memories of the trauma are not entirely forgotten. Trauma theorists speak of "body memory," a concept which underscores that even if the mind forgets, the body remembers. They note that some survivors have physical pains or sensations that result from unresolved memories and feelings about their traumas. For example, Bloom tells the story of a rape survivor who, years after her assault, began to suffer from chronic pelvic pain. Such physical symptoms are body memories or flashbacks—ways in which the body re-experiences past traumas, even if the mind does not consciously remember these events.[89]

For some trauma victims, this bodily nature of traumatic memory makes it seem as if their body has "turned against them."[90] As a result, many survivors—particularly abuse survivors—experience a sense of disconnection from their bodies. Some cope with this by attempting to change their body to gain control over it or to alter the way others view them.[91] They may develop eating disorders, dress in ways that conceal their shape, or make other changes to their appearance. Brison, for example, reports that after her attack she wished that she could put eyes in the back of her head; instead, she settled for a short haircut that made her look more like a man.[92] Sometimes, victims alter their appearance in an effort to become less attractive and thus less vulnerable to attack.[93]

FRAGMENTATION OF LANGUAGE

In addition to having fragmented memories, some trauma survivors experience a fracturing of language that invokes profound feelings of alienation. They find it difficult to write or speak about their traumas, sometimes even in the presence of those whom they love and trust. Some trauma scholars contend that this loss of language may happen because the brain stores traumatic memories in visual or sensory categories rather than in verbal-linguistic ones.[94] When memories are stored in this way, survivors may not consciously remember them and thus remain unable to describe them verbally. In other instances, survivors can recall their traumas but find that their memories have a "frozen and wordless quality" that lacks verbal narrative and context.[95] Bloom and Reichert describe this as similar to watching a movie without sound: The survivor mentally views the picture but does not have the words to articulate what happens in the scene.[96] Lodged in the body, traumatic memories have an unmediated quality that makes them difficult to symbolize in language.[97]

Holocaust survivor Primo Levi proposes a second reason that survivors may find it difficult to speak of their traumatic experiences. Instead of focusing on the nature of traumatic memory, Levi points to the limitations of language. He argues that the ongoing trauma which Jews experienced during the Holocaust was so horrible that language cannot adequately describe it. Levi claims that in everyday life,

> We say "hunger," we say "tiredness," "fear"' "pain," we say "winter". . . . [These] are free words, created and used by free men who lived in comfort and suffer-

> ing in their homes. If the Lagers had lasted longer a new, harsh language would have been born; and only this language could express what it means to toil the whole day in the wind, with the temperature below freezing, wearing only a shirt, underpants, cloth jacket and trousers, and in one's body nothing but weakness, hunger and knowledge of the end drawing nearer.[98]

For some survivors, language lacks the words to express their pain.

Susan Brison, a survivor of sexual assault and attempted murder, suggests a third reason that some traumatized people remain unable to speak of their experiences: Other people refuse to hear them. To create narratives of their traumas, survivors need not only the words with which to tell their stories, but also an empathic other who will listen to them. When people respond with empathy and compassion, survivors have the motivation and support they need to tell their stories.[99] However, when others respond with judgment, disbelief, or indifference—or when they simply refuse to listen at all—survivors can be retraumatized. It becomes difficult for them to tell their stories, even to themselves.[100] This leaves survivors feeling isolated and alone.

DIMINISHED AGENCY AND LOSS OF CONTROL

The disruptions in memory and language that trauma sometimes engenders can lead survivors to experience diminished agency, a loss of a sense of control over oneself and one's environment.[101] During a trauma people feel radically out of control: overwhelmed, speechless, shocked, and unable to defend themselves. For many survivors, this sense of being out of control continues in the aftermath of the trauma, as they contend with the knowledge that if tragedy happened once it may strike again.

Some trauma theorists argue that this loss of control is an especially crippling effect of trauma because human beings need a sense of control to function well in the world. According to Janoff-Bulman, most of us know on a conscious level that we cannot completely determine the direction of our lives and that sometimes things happen that we cannot predict or prevent. Yet on a deeper level, at the very core of our being, we tend to believe that we are in control of what happens to us. This conviction serves an important function: It enables us to go about out daily lives without being overwhelmed by all the things that could go radically wrong.[102]

For some survivors, the loss of control becomes more entrenched as they struggle with the ongoing effects of their traumas. Hyperarousal and intrusive memories reaffirm the "out of control" feeling because these responses happen against the victim's will and are hard to stop. In addition, individuals who continually dissociate in the face of stressful events may feel powerless to assess their immediate and long-term options and to choose actions that enable them to flourish. Moreover, some survivors lose control not only over their physiological responses, but also over their motivation to perform activities they previously had enjoyed. Brison gives the example of a sexual assault survivor whose fear of being assaulted again has taken away her desire to go for walks. Trauma, she explains, can both restrict what the survivor can do and limit what they want to do.[103]

In some instances, the survivor's loss of agency and control leads them to blame themselves for their traumas. Paradoxically, self-blame is one way to regain a sense of agency or control after a trauma: If we assume responsibility for what has happened to us, then we imply that we are, at least to some degree, able to control what happens to us. In this regard, self-blame is not merely a maladaptive response to trauma, but one that can help facilitate recovery by restoring to the victim some sense of agency and control. Janoff-Bulman contends that this is more likely to happen when victims blame their past, supposedly problematic (but presumably modifiable) behaviors for their misfortune, rather than their (presumably unmodifiable) character. Finding fault with one's character often leads over time to depression and a loss of self-esteem.[104]

Even though behavioral self-blame can function as an effective coping mechanism, it comes with certain costs. Brison contends that it may lead some survivors to berate themselves for past "mistakes" and to engage in "unfair, and ultimately futile, self-imposed restrictions on [their] behavior."[105] In addition, behavioral self-blame reinforces society's harmful tendency to find fault with victims for what has happened to them.[106] Those who do not experience traumas firsthand often blame survivors to protect their own sense that if only they do the right things, they can keep such horrible events from happening to them. And so they may say, for example, that a woman was attacked because she dressed the wrong way or walked alone at night. In other words, she was in control and could have prevented the assault.

While trauma survivors sometimes lose a sense of agency and control, they also often successfully assert their agency in creative and daring ways, both during the trauma and in its aftermath. For example, domestic violence survivors who call the police, seek help from a shelter, or confide in a trusted friend are exercising their agency. Similarly, an abused woman who laughs when her perpetrator gives her orders is asserting her autonomy and refusing to relinquish complete control.[107] As Evan Stark observes, clinical trauma theory has tended to emphasize the victimization of trauma survivors in ways that obscure their resilience and strength. While it is clear that trauma can lead to psychological disintegration, many traumatized persons boldly resist this disintegration, sometimes at great personal cost, by openly or subtly defying the perpetrators who seek to "co-opt and deconstruct [their] personhood."[108] What often results in situations of trauma is thus a dynamic interplay of agency and victimization, a complex struggle that renders traumatized persons not pure victims but rather both victims and survivors.[109]

LOSS OF A TEMPORAL TIMELINE

Along with the loss of control, some trauma survivors experience a loss of ability to construct a temporal timeline of events and experiences that constitute their life stories. The insights of trauma scholars suggest that having a sense of a temporal timeline that incorporates experiences from our past, present, and future is essential to our identities. Human beings derive meaning and a sense of our own value partly from the stories we remember and tell about our lives, and it gives us a sense of internal integration when we can place these stories into a broader, overarching narrative that spans from the past into the future. But some trauma survivors lack this sense of temporal timeline, for several reasons. First, dissociation can lead them to experience gaps in their memory that make it hard to recall specific incidents or whole periods of time.

Second, intrusive memories and hyperarousal can blur the distinction between past and present. When traumatized people relive their traumas through hyperarousal or memory disruptions, they feel as though their traumatic past is intruding into the present, such that it is not really "past" at all. When this happens, the trauma takes on a totalizing force: It overwhelms the survivor and becomes the sole focus of their thoughts and energy. To put it differently, trauma can narrow the survivor's perspective, rendering their vision myopic so that they dwell on their traumatic experience. Stuck in the moment of trauma, he or she does not feel as though time flows smoothly and continuously from the past into the future. Instead, the traumatic past overwhelms the present and, from the survivor's perspective, defines the whole of his or her life.

The myopic vision that can result from trauma restricts the victim's imaginative capacities, undermining the individual's ability to develop a positive vision for the future. When people get stuck in a traumatic moment, the future—to the extent that they can think about it at all—looks bleak indeed. Some survivors imagine that life will always be as hard as it is now; as a result, they find it difficult to construct plans and goals for who they want to become and what they want to achieve. Survivors who contend on a daily basis with trauma symptoms may lack the emotional energy necessary to reflect on their goals and dreams. Others can think about the future but envision it in profoundly negative ways, partly because their past traumatic experiences have led them to develop a pessimistic worldview. Instead of showing them that the world is benevolent and that good things will happen, their traumatic experiences have taught them to believe that life is unfair, the world is cruel, and people should not be trusted.[110]

SHATTERED SELF-CONCEPT

Trauma scholars often suggest that a strong, healthy sense of our identity and goodness is essential to living a productive and happy life. To have a sense of coherence and stable relationships with others, human beings need to believe in our abilities and to see ourselves as worthy of love and attention. Trauma, however, can undermine such positive self-perceptions. It can damage self-respect and, in some instances, lead to self-loathing, shame, guilt, and a sense of inadequacy.[111] For example, physical abuse survivors may experience negative emotions that stem from the damage done to their bodies, which makes them feel violated. As Brison notes, people who commit such abuse treat their victims as "mere flesh": "It is as if the tormentor says with his blows, 'You are nothing but a body, a mere object for my will—here, I'll prove it!'"[112] Being reduced to a body reinforces feelings of powerlessness and incompetence—feelings that many abusers underscore by verbally degrading or scapegoating their victims.[113]

Trauma damages the survivor's self-perceptions most severely when the abuse is repeated. As Herman notes, "While the victim of the single acute trauma may feel after the event that she is 'not herself,' the victim of chronic trauma may . . . lose the sense that she has any self at all."[114] In some instances, victims never develop this sense of self in the first place. Herman observes that for many children who suffer chronic abuse, "fragmentation becomes the central principle of personality organization."[115] Faced with the impossible task of coping with overwhelming experiences before their psychological defenses are fully formed, traumatized children often do not develop the sense of inner safety and independence that would help them to construct an integrated identity.

THE FRACTURING OF RELATIONSHIPS

The description of traumatization offered so far has focused largely on the psychological consequences of trauma. But trauma is not just a psychological phenomenon. While the *DSM*'s diagnostic criteria for post-traumatic stress disorder concentrate on several core individual psychological symptoms—persistently re-experiencing the trauma through intrusive memories, dreams, and flashbacks; increased arousal; and avoidance of trauma-related stimuli—many trauma theorists recognize that trauma can have a much broader range of effects.[116] It cannot only lead to psychological symptoms but also have social, spiritual, and relational consequences. Specifically, trauma can change how people view and interact with other people and God. To develop a more complete account of trauma's effects, then, requires addressing the questions: What kinds of interpersonal relationships do traumatized people tend to seek? How do their traumas affect their current relationships? Moreover, how does trauma shape people's images of God and their experiences of religious communities?

Trauma and Human Relationships

Trauma survivors have different experiences with interpersonal relationships after their traumas. For some survivors, interpersonal relationships function as a positive force in their healing process. They draw strength from the support of family and friends, or develop new friendships that help them to cope in healthy ways. Other survivors, however, experience problems with relationships that can take two different forms. First, they may have trouble forming or sustaining stable relationships, possibly because they experience emotional numbing that makes it difficult to feel the love and empathy which deep friendships require; or, because they have lost their basic trust in people and thus refrain from seeking close relationships for fear of being harmed again.[117] In addition, survivors may feel guilt, shame, fear, or a sense of inferiority that causes them to minimize their participation in social life.[118] Sometimes, traumatized people fail to see a connection between their traumas and their relational difficulties. They know that they are having a hard time with relationships but do not understand why.[119]

Second, other survivors find that their traumas cause them to seek unhealthy attachments to others. An especially harmful pattern is "trauma bonding," when survivors attach to their perpetrators.[120] Particularly common among abused children and adult torture victims, trauma bonding takes place partly because the offender functions as the victims' only source for survival and hope. In such situations, victims may attach to this person because they become utterly dependent on him or her. As a result, the perpetrator gains psychological as well as physical control, and feelings of helplessness come to dominate the survivor's internal world.[121]

The deep desire for attachment can make survivors particularly vulnerable to revictimization. As they seek to forge new relationships, survivors may turn to individuals who do not have their best interests at heart. For example, people who were abused as children are more likely to become involved in relationships in which they are mistreated as adults.[122] In some instances, survivors crave attachments but have internalized a deep sense of inferiority as a result of their abuse, which leads them to become involved in relationships of dependence in which they have little power and respect. In other cases, survivors are at risk for revictimization because their coping mechanisms, such as hyperarousal and dissociation, prevent them from perceiving external or internal cues that would warn them of danger. According to Herman, trauma survivors do not actively seek revictimization; rather, they tend to experience it "as a dreaded but unavoidable fate. . . . Many survivors have such profound deficiencies in self-protection that they can barely imagine themselves in a position of agency or choice."[123]

Trauma and Religion

As Carolyn Yoder observes, human beings are meaning-making creatures.[124] Our sense of safety and stability depends on our ability to find meaning in the world and in the events that constitute our life stories. As creatures who crave meaning, we want to believe that things happen for a reason and that the world is fair and predictable. This search for meaning—for explanation and for a sense of purpose—is a spiritual quest that leads many people to belief in the divine. For some, this belief is defined by communal creeds and practices; for others it remains more individual, amorphous, or evolving.

Trauma challenges people's ability to find meaning in the world. In the aftermath of a traumatic experience, it is common for survivors to doubt that their lives have a purpose and that the world has any meaning at all. For those who normally turn to religion as a way to find meaning, trauma may pose an especially difficult challenge by raising troubling theological questions: Why doesn't God stop such terrible things from happening? What kind of a God allows people to suffer violence and abuse? Does everything really happen for a reason—and if so, what reason could there possibly be for trauma? Is it possible to make sense out of traumatic violence? Trauma forces many survivors to rethink their fundamental convictions about the divine. Precisely how they reconsider these convictions, however, varies from one person to the next.

While some survivors do not experience a change in their views of God, others report that their traumas have led them to feel more negatively toward God. For example, some feel shame before God. Others fear God (whom they view as cruel) or feel abandoned by God.[125] As one incest survivor says, "I was wondering where was God when I was being abused? I mean he totally ignored me as a child."[126] A combat veteran describes his loss of faith in this way:

> I could not rationalize in my mind how God let good men die. I had gone to several . . . priests. I was sitting there with this one priest and said, "Father, I don't understand this. . . . I got all these friends who are dead." . . . That priest, he looked me in the eye and said, "I don't know, son, I've never been in war." I said, "I didn't ask you about war, I asked you about God"[127]

Traumatized people emphasize the themes of God's absence, silence, and distance more than non-traumatized people.[128] In addition, they often express intense feelings of unworthiness before God, as well as a loss of trust in and anger at God.[129]

Some trauma theorists argue that these negative effects of trauma on survivors' relationships with God stems from a correlation between one's images of others and one's images of the divine. Although they differ in their understandings of precisely how one's perceptions of God are created, many trauma theorists contend that early in childhood, children form an image of God based partly on their image of their parents. Thus, if a child perceives her parents to be benevolent and kind, she comes to view God as even more benevolent and kind than her mother and father.[130] While some trauma theorists focus exclusively on the parents' role in the formation of the child's God-image, another theory holds that the child's relationships with her entire family—and with others outside of the family—also shape her perceptions of divine attitudes and behaviors.[131]

Carrie Doehring argues that this God-image formed early in childhood does not necessarily remain static over the course of one's life. More specifically, she contends that experiencing severe childhood or adolescent abuse leads some individuals to express more negative views of God as adults than those who have not been deeply traumatizated.[132] Given the correlation between our God-images and our social relationships, this is not surprising. Traumatized persons may perceive God as more wrathful, angry, and punitive than others because this is precisely how they have experienced their perpetrators. Note, however, that this correlation between social relationships and relationships with God may not be unilinear. Doehring proposes that it has a bi-directional character: Just as traumatic stressors can shape one's God image, so one's views of God can shape how one responds to traumatic stressors.[133]

Sheila Redmond, a therapist who works with trauma survivors, offers one perspective on how a person's view of God can shape his or her response to trauma. Based on her work with child abuse survivors from Christian backgrounds, Redmond argues that some traumatized persons do not perceive a change in their religious views because they suppress the spiritual effects of their traumas. This suppression happens because they receive a view of God from their families and churches that they find difficult to reconcile with their traumas: God as "a loving father, a punishing father, an all-knowing father, an all-seeing father, an all-powerful father. . . . Everything is under his control."[134] Often, survivors cannot understand why this benevolent and all-powerful God allows their suffering. To resolve this contradiction, they blame themselves for their traumas. It is easier to believe they have done something wrong than to figure out why God permits their abuse. Unfortunately, this self-blame can be debilitating, as survivors grow increasingly convinced of their guilt, worthlessness, and inherent badness.[135]

Along with their conflicted relationships with God, many trauma survivors have negative experiences with religious communities and their practices. Some feel betrayed by these communities, which failed to protect them; many abusers come from families active in religious organizations, and many abuse survivors come from "model" religious homes.[136] In other instances, survivors experience a loss of trust in faith communities because these communities actively participated in their abuse, as in cases of clergy sexual misconduct. In addition, survivors who are harmed outside of religious communities may have negative experiences in these communities because they use practices, symbols, and beliefs that play upon survivors' traumas, reinvoking traumatic memories and feelings of anxiety or depression. For example, some survivors who grew up in Christian contexts note the ways in which specific doctrines, such as original sin and the need for redemption, reinforce their feelings of guilt and self-blame.[137] Christian feminist theologians also point out how images of violence used in religious settings—such as the symbol of the cross that remains central to Christian liturgy and preaching—may trigger traumatic flashbacks.[138] For some trauma survivors, hearing about Jesus' violent death in a sermon or seeing this symbol displayed over the altar can bring back painful memories of the survivor's own violent traumatic experiences.[139]

In other situations, trauma survivors feel negatively toward faith communities that did not actively perpetrate violent harm but failed to provide narratives, symbols, or practices that could address their needs for healing. Some traumatized people turn to religious groups for support and are disappointed when they do not find helpful resources there. One survivor who has actively participated in Christian communities over the course of her life says, "I have always sought answers in the church for how to get healed from all this stuff. I expected to find it there and never did. . . . When I realized that the church had never helped me, I felt a real letdown. It was disappointing; it made me angry because the church should be one place you find the promise of healing."[140]

Not all survivors, however, have negative experiences of religious groups. Some find social support in such communities and consider them crucial to the preservation of their identity.[141] According to McFarlane and van der Kolk, some survivors claim that the rituals and practices of their religious communities help them to overcome their isolation by connecting them with the suffering of others, both past and present.[142] Other traumatized people find that their participation in religious communities gives them hope and sustenance by offering a framework through which they address questions of meaning and overcome their sense of forsakenness by God and other people. I explore this complex relation between traumatic violence, religion, and meaning-making in chapters 5 and 6, when I offer theological reflections on trauma and nonviolence.

THE TRAUMATIZED SELF

What, finally, is the picture of the traumatized self that emerges from trauma scholars' descriptions of traumatic violence? At a most basic level, trauma theorists portray the traumatized self as a severely fragmented self, which has a fractured sense of self and world. "Traumatized people," Herman says, "suffer damage to the basic structures of the self. They lose their trust in themselves, in other people, and in God. Their self-esteem is assaulted. . . . Their capacity for intimacy is compromised. . . . The identity they have formed prior to the trauma is irrevocably destroyed."[143]

In describing the long-term effects of trauma in this way, trauma theorists suggest that the traumatized self can become a site of violence, in which the experience of traumatic violence is repeatedly replayed and reenacted. As we have seen, trauma survivors can experience this repetition in numerous ways: for example, through flashbacks, intrusive memories, nightmares, hyperarousal, and behavioral reenactments of their traumas. According to Serene Jones, trauma theorists indicate that survivors who endure these ongoing effects of trauma often come to experience themselves as imprisoned within a traumatic reality.[144] Unlike other prisons, however, the barriers that constrain them operate not from the outside but from within. Experiencing this imprisonment over a prolonged time deepens the fracturing or fragmentation of the survivor's self.

This picture of the traumatized self as deeply fragmented both resonates with and differs from other contemporary descriptions of the fragmented self. In particular, poststructuralist theorists speak of the self's fragmentation; indeed, they have undertaken the very project of "decentering the subject." Unlike trauma theorists, however, poststructuralists see this fragmentation or decentering as something to be celebrated; for them, it refers to the dismantling of gender essentialisms underlying Western thought that lock men and women into stereotypical gender roles. From a poststructuralist perspective, the self is not a stable entity, but rather is thoroughly constituted in and through the "discursive and social relations" of its culture.[145] Poststructuralists' attempt to describe this constitution—to de-stabilize the subject—offers insight into our sexist cultural patterns and the ways we are, in fact, products of our environments.

While poststructuralist understandings of the fragmented self make an important theoretical contribution, they overlook a crucial insight of trauma studies: Human beings need a certain core sense of self to function well in the world.[146] The very fragmentation that poststructuralists applaud represents a condition or state of being that trauma theorists see as profoundly harmful and debilitating.[147] The insights of trauma scholars suggest that the self's fragmentation must not be celebrated but rather transformed. More specifically, the traumatized self does not need more fragmentation, but an ongoing process of healing that reintegrates the self, giving it a basic wholeness or coherence.[148]

Unlike poststructuralists, trauma scholars thus articulate a normative vision of the self. More specifically, they speak in ways which indicate that for selves to successfully negotiate their way through the world, they need to have a few capacities or features, such as agency, relationality, ordered memory, embodiment, and language. The potential for these capacities is present in all human beings from birth, and the development or actualization of them over time is necessary for the self to be a healthy, well-functioning self. They are not, however, impervious to our engagement with culture and history. While these features of the self cannot be completely accounted for as cultural productions, they are nonetheless profoundly shaped—and sometimes diminished or destroyed—by our social contexts.

Even as trauma scholars emphasize the wholeness and coherence that non-traumatized selves enjoy, they often acknowledge that given the multiple dimensions of selfhood, all persons experience some degree of fragmentation.[149] But their work suggests that despite this fragmentation, the healthy self has a certain integrity: its features remain intact. This "intactness" is precisely what enables it to perform many of its basic patterns of daily functioning. For example, selves that are whole or coherent can act as intentional agents, establish solid interpersonal relationships, feel physically safe in their surroundings, and create ongoing personal narratives of particular events and experiences. It is precisely these abilities that trauma can strip away over time as it moves from the outside in.

As we have seen, the fragmentation that trauma scholars describe is not a condition that all persons experience but one that results specifically from overwhelming violence that moves into the self, making it a site of violence. This image of the self as a site of violence has implications for Christian nonviolence: It implies that trauma is part of the identity and life of the church, which is partially constituted by traumatized persons. As noted, this does not mean that trauma has an impact only on those persons who have directly endured it. Since the church is a social organism in which what affects one member also affects the others (albeit in different ways), trauma is a reality with which the entire church body must contend.

Trauma studies thus encourages Christians to think more expansively about what it means to communally practice nonviolence. Understanding nonviolence as the refusal to act as an agent of violence is a start, but it must entail more than this. Christian nonviolence must also include working to resist and transform internalized, traumatic violence. It must entail contributing to the healing of selves that are sites of violence by creating a space in which traumatized persons can survive and flourish.

Since the church has perpetrated violence in many ways throughout history, it is hard to say precisely how Christian communities can create such spaces and what they would look like. One way to get some traction on this matter, however, is to explore what trauma scholars say about healing from trauma. In the next chapter I undertake this task, summarizing some of their most central insights. This lays the theoretical foundation for the final three chapters of the book, in which I bring these insights into conversation with Christian theology to consider how the church might enact nonviolence as the healing or transformation of internalized, traumatic violence.

NOTES

1. Terr, *Too Scared to Cry: How Trauma Affects Children and Ultimately Us All* (New York: Basic Books, 1990), 13–26, 170–71, 211–13.

2. For example, see Susan Brison, *Aftermath: Violence and the remaking of a self* (Princeton: Princeton University Press, 2000); Flora Keshgegian, *Redeeming Memories*; Jennifer Beste, *God and the Victim*; and Mary E. Gilfus, "The Price of a Ticket."

3. Ruth Leys, *Trauma: A Genealogy* (Chicago: The University of Chicago Press, 2000), 3.

4. Leys, *Trauma: A Genealogy*, 3–4.

5. Leys, *Trauma: A Genealogy*, 4.

6. Herman, *Trauma and Recovery* (New York: BasicBooks, 1992), 26–28. Obviously, interest in trauma and posttraumatic stress disorder has peaked again due to the war in Iraq.

7. For instance, see Judith Herman's classic text, *Trauma and Recovery*.

8. See Bessel A. van der Kolk, "The Body Keeps the Score: Approaches to the Psychobiology of Posttraumatic Stress Disorder," in *Traumatic Stress: The Effects of Overwhelming Experience on Mind, Body, and Society*, eds. van der Kolk, Alexander C. McFarlane, and Lars Weisaeth (New York: Guilford Press, 1996).

9. See James Young, *Writing and Rewriting the Holocaust: Narrative and the Consequences of Interpretation* (Bloomington: Indiana University Press, 1988), and Karl Plank, *Mother of the Wire Fence: Inside and Outside the Holocaust* (Louisville, KY: Westminster John Knox Press, 1994).

10. See Martha Minow, *Between Vengeance and Forgiveness: Facing History after Genocide* (Boston: Beacon Press, 1998) and Herbert Hirsch, *Genocide and the Politics of Memory: Studying Death to Preserve Life* (Chapel Hill: University of North Carolina Press, 1995).

11. See Nell Painter, *Soul Murder and Slavery* (Waco: Markham Press Fund, Baylor University Press, 1995) and Saidiya Hartman, *Scenes of Subjection: Terror, Slavery, and Self-Making in Nineteenth-Century America* (New York: Oxford University Press, 1997).

12. *Unclaimed Experience: Trauma, Narrative, and History* (Baltimore: The Johns Hopkins University Press, 1996), 3.

13. *Unclaimed Experience*, 3.

14. For example, see van der Kolk and McFarlane, "The Black Hole of Trauma," in *Traumatic Stress: The Effects of Overwhelming Experience on Mind, Body, and Society*, eds., Bessel A. van der Kolk, Alexander C. McFarlane, and Lars Weisaeth (New York: Guilford Press, 1996), 6.

15. Van der Kolk and McFarlane, "The Black Hole of Trauma," *Traumatic Stress*, 6.

16. Van der Kolk and McFarlane, "The Black Hole of Trauma," 7.

17. Van der Kolk and McFarlane, "The Black Hole of Trauma," 5.

18. Van der Kolk and McFarlane, "The Black Hole of Trauma," 8.

19. Van der Kolk and McFarlane, "The Black Hole of Trauma," 6.

20. Cathy Caruth, *Trauma and Memory* (Baltimore: Johns Hopkins University Press, 1995), 5.

21. Maria P. P. Root, "Reconstructing the Impact of Trauma on Personality," in *Personality and Psychopathology: Feminist Reappraisals*, eds. Laura S. Brown and Mary Ballou (New York: The Guilford Press, 1992), 37.

22. Herman, *Trauma and Recovery*, 58.

23. Jennifer Beste discusses these four categories in *God and the Victim: Traumatic Intrusions on Grace and Freedom* (New York: Oxford University Press, 2007), 6–8. Other scholars break them down into six distinct categories. See van der Kolk, *Psychological Trauma* (Washington, DC: American Psychiatric Press, 1987), and Carrie Doehring, *Internal Desecration* (Lanham, MD: University Press of America, 1993), 2–5.

24. See Alexander McFarlane, "The Nature of Traumatic Stressors and the Epidemiology of Posttraumatic Reactions," in *Traumatic Stress*, 130; Jon G. Allen, *Coping with Trauma: A Guide to Self-Understanding* (Washington, DC: American Psychiatric Press, Inc., 1995), 5–13.

25. *Diagnostic and Statistical Manual of Mental Disorders: DSM-IV*, Washington, DC: American Psychiatric Association, 1994, 424–29.

26. This distinction can become blurred in the case of disasters such as nuclear accidents, gasoline spills, and toxic poisonings that are the result of human actions. See Kai Erikson, *A New Species of Trouble* (New York: W.W. Norton & Company, 1994).

27. Jeffrey Means and Mary Ann Nelson, *Trauma and Evil: Healing the Wounded Soul* (Minneapolis: Fortress Press, 2000), 67.

28. For example, see Means and Nelson, *Trauma and Evil*, 67–68.

29. "Stress versus Traumatic Stress: From Acute Homeostatic Reactions to Chronic Psychopathology," in *Traumatic Stress*, 87.

30. Shalev, "Stress versus Traumatic Stress," 87.

31. Marten W. DeVries, "Trauma in Cultural Perspective," in *Traumatic Stress*, 404.

32. McFarlane and van der Kolk, "Trauma and Its Challenge to Society,", 29–30.

33. McFarlane and van der Kolk, "Trauma and Its Challenge to Society," 25.

34. Janoff-Bulman, *Shattered Assumptions: Towards a New Psychology of Trauma* (New York: The Free Press, 1992), 147–57.

35. "Trauma and Its Challenge to Society," 25.

36. McFarlane and van der Kolk, "Trauma and Its Challenge to Society," 39.

37. *Diagnostic and Statistical Manual of Mental Disorder: DSM-III* (Washington, DC: American Psychiatric Association, 1980). The 1952 edition did, however, include a

category of traumatic neurosis that provided a foundation for PTSD. See *Diagnostic and Statistical Manual of Mental Disorder* (Washington, DC: American Psychiatric Association, 1952).

38. *Diagnostic and Statistical Manual of Mental Disorders: DSM-III* (Washington, DC: American Psychiatric Associaton, 1980), 236.

39. See Diana E. H. Russell and Rebecca M. Bolen, *The Epidemic of Rape and Child Sexual Abuse* (Thousand Oaks, CA: Sage Publications, 2000); Pamela Cooper-White, *The Cry of Tamar: Violence Against Women and the Church's Response* (Minneapolis: Augsburg Fortress Press, 1995), 152; Anthony Urquiza and Lisa Marie Keating, "The Prevalence of Sexual Victimization in Males," in *The Sexually Abused Male*, ed. Mic Hunter (New York: Lexington Books, 1990).

40. Jennifer Manlowe, *Faith Born of Seduction: Sexual Trauma, Body Image, and Religion* (New York: New York University Press, 1995), 1.

41. Herman, *Trauma and Recovery*, 33.

42. See Mary E. Gilfus, "The Price of a Ticket"; Maria P. P. Root, "Reconstructing the Impact of Trauma on Personality," 229–61; and Laura S. Brown, "Not Outside the Range: One Feminist Perspective on Psychic Trauma," 100–112.

43. Gilfus, "The Price of a Ticket," 1243.

44. Gilfus, "The Price of a Ticket," 1243.

45. Gilfus, "The Price of a Ticket," 1241; Brown, "Not Outside the Range," 102.

46. Gilfus, "The Price of a Ticket," 1242.

47. Brown, "Not Outside the Range," 107; Root, "Reconstructing the Impact of Trauma on Personality," 240.

48. Root, "Reconstructing the Impact of Trauma on Personality," 240; Brown, "Not Outside the Range," 105.

49. Root, "Reconstructing the Impact of Trauma on Personality," 239–40.

50. See Lori Hope Lefkovitz, "Inherited Holocaust Memory and the Ethics of Ventriloquism," *The Kenyon Review* ns 19 (Winter 1997): 34–43 and Karein Goertz, "Transgenerational Representations of the Holocaust: From Memory to Post-Memory," *World Literature Today* 72:1 (Winter 1998): 33–38.

51. Brown, "Not Outside the Range," 107–8.

52. Brown, "Not Outside the Range," 107–8.

53. Alexander C. McFarlane and Giovanni de Girolamo, "The Nature of Traumatic Stressors and the Epidemiology of Posttraumatic Reactions," in *Traumatic Stress*, 129.

54. McFarlane and Girolamo, "The Nature of Traumatic Stressors," 130.

55. Sandra Bloom and Michael Reichert, *Bearing Witness: Violence and Collective Responsibility* (New York: The Haworth Maltreatment and Trauma Press, 1998), 116.

56. Van der Kolk and McFarlane, "The Black Hole of Trauma," 6.

57. Van der Kolk and McFarlane, "The Black Hole of Trauma," 13.

58. Van der Kolk, "The Body Keeps the Score: Approaches to the Psychobiology of Posttraumatic Stress Disorder," in *Traumatic Stress*, 219. See also Ronnie Janoff-Bulman, *Shattered Assumptions: Towards a New Psychology of Trauma* (New York: The Free Press, 1992), 65–69.

59. Van der Kolk, "The Psychobiology of PTSD," in *Traumatic Stress*, 218–219.

60. Janoff-Bulman, *Shattered Assumptions*, 68.

61. Herman, *Trauma and Recovery*, 108.

62. Herman, *Trauma and Recovery*, 35–36; Janoff-Bulman, *Shattered Assumptions*, 65.

63. Janoff-Bulman, *Shattered Assumptions,* 65.

64. Janoff-Bulman, *Shattered Assumptions,* 64.

65. Van der Kolk and McFarlane, "The Black Hole of Trauma," 12. Ronnie Janoff-Bulman notes that trauma theorists do not agree on whether this is a conscious or unconscious process. *Shattered Assumptions,* 96.

66. H. Krystal, *Massive Psychic Trauma* (New York: International Universities Press,) qtd. in van der Kolk, McFarlane, and van der Hart, "A General Approach to Treatment," in *Traumatic Stress,* 422.

67. Herman, *Trauma and Recovery,* 47.

68. Janoff-Bulman, *Shattered Assumptions,* 95–96.

69. Janoff-Bulman, *Shattered Assumptions,* 95.

70. Eve B. Carlson, Judith Armstrong, Richard Loewenstein, and David Roth, "Relationships Between Traumatic Experiences and Symptoms of Posttraumatic Stress, Dissociation, and Amnesia," in *Trauma, Memory, and Dissociation,* eds. J. Douglas Bremner and Charles R. Marmar (Washington, DC: American Psychiatric Press, Inc., 1998), 205–7.

71. The *DSM-IV* specifies that a diagnosis of PTSD requires that the three key trauma symptoms discussed so far—increased arousal, avoidance, and reexperiencing the trauma—be present for more than one month, and "the disturbance must cause clinically significant distress or impairment in social, occupational, or other important areas of functioning," 424.

72. Bessel van der Kolk, Onno van der Hart, and Charles R. Marmar, "Dissociation and Information Processing in PTSD," in *Traumatic Stress,* p. 306. See also Janoff-Bulman, *Shattered Assumptions,* 101.

73. See Bloom and Reichert, *Bearing Witness,* 124.

74. Bessel van der Kolk, Onno van der Hart, and Charles Marmar, "Dissociation and Informating Processing in PTSD," 307. Janoff-Bulman notes that many psychologists think of the most severe cases of dissociation as those that include the formation of split-off personality fragments called "alters" (formerly "multiple personalities"). See Janoff-Bulman, *Shattered Assumptions,* 102.

75. Janoff-Bulman, *Shattered Assumptions,* 102.

76. Janoff-Bulman, *Shattered Assumptions,* 103.

77. Bloom and Reichert, *Bearing Witness,* 114–15, and van der Kolk, "Trauma and Memory," in *Traumatic Stress,* 279–302.

78. See L. Squire, *Memory and the Brain* (New York: Oxford University Press, 1987) and van der Kolk, "Trauma and Memory," in *Traumatic Stress,* 280–281.

79. Bloom, *Creating Sanctuary: Toward an Evolution of Sane Societies* (New York: Routledge, 1997), 27.

80. Bloom and Reichert, *Bearing Witness,* 114–15.

81. Bloom, *Creating Sanctuary,* 26–27.

82. See Bloom and Reichert, *Bearing Witness,* 115.

83. Van der Kolk, "Trauma and Memory," 286–87; Herman, *Trauma and Recovery,* 38.

84. Van der Kolk, "Trauma and Memory," 287.

85. Van der Kolk, McFarlane, and van der Hart, "A General Approach to Treatment," in *Traumatic Stress,* 422; Brison, *Aftermath,* 15.

86. Brison, *Aftermath,* 32.

87. Kirmayer, "Landscapes of Memory," in *Tense Past: Cultural Essays in Trauma and* Memory, eds. Paul Antze and Michael Lambek (New York: Routledge, 1996), 188.

88. Kirmayer, "Landscapes of Memory," 189–90.

89. Bloom and Reichert, *Bearing Witness*, 117. Brison notes that people can have flashbacks of nontraumatic experiences as well, but these flashbacks occur without the painful emotions and physiological effects that accompany traumatic memories. *Aftermath*, *45*.

90. Herman, *Trauma and Recovery*, 86.

91. Brison, *Aftermath*, 46.

92. Brison, *Aftermath*, 46.

93. On the relationship between sexual trauma and eating disorders, see Jennifer L. Manlowe, *Faith Born of Seduction*; A. Abramson and G. Lucido, "Childhood Sexual Experience and Bulimia," *Addictive Behaviors* 16 (1991): 529–32; R. Palmer, et al., "Childhood Sexual Experiences with Adults Reported by Women with Eating Disorders: An Extended Series," *British Journal of Psychiatry* 156 (1990): 669–703; Maria P. P. Root and P. Fallon, "Persistent, Disordered Eating as a Gender Specific, Post-Traumatic Stress Response to Sexual Assault," *Psychotherapy* 28, no. 1 (Spring 1991): 96–104.

94. For example, see van der Kolk, "Trauma and Memory," 279–302; and Herman, *Trauma and Recovery*, 175.

95. Herman, *Trauma and Recovery*, 37.

96. Bloom and Reichert, *Bearing Witness*, 116.

97. van der Kolk, "Trauma and Memory," 287.

98. Levi, *Survival in Auschwitz* (New York: Collier Books, 1961), 112–13.

99. Brison, *Aftermath*, 51. See also Dori Laub, ""Bearing Witness or the Vicissitudes of Listening," in *Testimony: Crises of Witnessing in Literature, Psychoanalysis, and History*, eds. Shoshana Felman and Dori Laub, M.D. (New York: Routledge, Chapman and Hall, Inc., 1992), 57–74; Laub, "An Event Without Witness: Truth, Testimony, and Survival," *Testimony*, 75–92; Levi, *Survival in Auschwitz*, 54.

100. Brison, *Aftermath*, 50.

101. In philosophical and ethical discourse, agency is often defined as the power or potentiality for action [See Maura A. Ryan, "Agency," in *Dictionary of Feminist Theologies*, eds. Letty M. Russell and Shannon Clarkson (Louisville, KY: Westminster John Knox Press, 1996), 4–5]. When trauma scholars say that survivors have lost agency, however, they do not mean that these individuals no longer have the power to act (although this power to act may be diminished in some instances, such as when they dissociate). Rather, they mean that survivors lose a sense of control over their responses and their lives. Thus, they experience a loss of what some ethicists and philosophers call "autonomous agency." For an extended account of trauma and agency, see Jennifer Beste, *God and the Victim*.

102. Janoff-Bulman, *Shattered Assumptions: Towards a New Psychology of Trauma* (New York: The Free Press, 1992).

103. Brison, *Aftermath*, 59–60.

104. Ronnie Janoff-Bulman, "Characterological versus Behavioral Self-Blame: Inquiries into Depression and Rape," *Journal of Personality and Social Psychology* 37, no. 10 (1979): 1798–1809.

105. Brison, *Aftermath*, 75–76.

106. Brison, *Aftermath*, 76.

107. Evan Stark gives this example in *Coercive Control: How Men Entrap Women in Personal Life* (New York: Oxford University Press, 2007), 215–16.

108. Stark, *Coercive Control*, 215.

109. See Stark, *Coercive Control*, 215–16.

110. See Ronnie Janoff-Bulman, *Shattered Assumptions*, 70–90.

111. Herman, *Trauma and Recovery*, 121.

112. Brison, *Aftermath*, 47.

113. Herman, *Trauma and Recovery*, 103–4.

114. Herman, *Trauma and Recovery*, 86.

115. Herman, *Trauma and Recovery*, 107.

116. Herman attempts to account for these additional effects by introducing the category of "complex posttraumatic stress disorder." See *Trauma and Recovery*, ch. 6. See also Herman, "Complex PTSD: A Syndrome in Survivors of Prolonged and Repeated Trauma," in *Psychotraumatology: Key Papers and Core Concepts in Post-traumatic Stress*, eds. George S. Everly, Jr., and Jeffrey M. Lating (New York: Plenum Press, 1995), 87–100. The *DSM-IV* also includes as "associated features and disorders" several other trauma symptoms, such as guilt, social withdrawal, feelings of inadequacy and hopelessness, impaired interpersonal relationships, and hostility.

117. Herman, *Trauma and Recovery*, 121.

118. Herman, *Trauma and Recovery*, 53–55; Brison, *Aftermath*, 60.

119. See James DeBoe, "Personality-Splitting Trauma," *Perspectives* 7 (September 1992): 13–15; Janoff-Bulman, *Shattered Assumptions*, 63.

120. See Bloom and Reichert, *Bearing Witness*, 139–140.

121. Herman, *Trauma and Recovery*, 81–82.

122. Herman, *Trauma and Recovery*, 113.

123. Herman, *Trauma and Recovery*, 112.

124. Yoder, *The Little Book of Trauma Healing: When Violence Strikes and Community Security Is Threatened* (Intercourse, PA: Good Books, Inc., 2005), 25.

125. See Jennifer Manlowe, *Faith Born of Seduction*, 83–84 ; John Stapert, "God Enters Dark Closets," *Perspectives* 7 (September 1992): 16–18; Kane, Cheston, and Greer, "Perception of God by Survivors of Childhood Sexual Abuse: An Exploratory Study in an Underresearched Area," *Journal of Psychology and Theology* 21 (1993): 228–37; Terese A. Hall, "Spiritual Effects of Childhood Sexual Abuse in Adult Christian Women," *Journal of Psychology and Theology* 23 (1995): 129–34.

126. Qtd. in Manlowe, *Faith Born of Seduction*, 83.

127. Qtd. in Herman, *Trauma and Recovery*, 55.

128. Kane, et al., "Perceptions of God by Survivors of Childhood Sexual Abuse," 228–37.

129. Kane, et al., "Perceptions of God by Survivors of Childhood Sexual Abuse," 228–37.

130. William G. Justice and Warren Lambert, "A Comparative Study of the Language People Use to Describe the Personalities of God and Their Earthly Parents," *The Journal of Pastoral Care* 40, no. 2 (June 1986): 166–72; John Lemoncelli and Andrew Carey, "The Psychospiritual Dynamics of Adult Survivors of Abuse," *Counseling and Values* 40:3 (1996): 175–84.

131. Ana-Maria Rizzuto, *Birth of the Living God: A Psychoanalytic Study* (Chicago: The University of Chicago Press, 1979).

132. Doehring, *Internal Desecration: Traumatization and Representations of God* (Lanham, MD: University Press of America, 1993).

133. See Doehring, *Internal Desecration*, 10.

134. Redmond, "God Died and Nobody Gave a Funeral," *Pastoral Psychology* 45, no. 1 (1996): 42–43.

135. Herman, *Trauma and Recovery*, 103–5.

136. Carino, "A Dark Room in My Mind," *Perspectives* 7 (September 1992): 9.

137. Redmond, "God Died," 44.

138. See Serene Jones, "Trauma and Grace," in *Reflections*, a magazine of the Yale Divinity School community and edited by Jamie L. Manson. Jones' article appears in the winter 2004 edition, 8–15.

139. See Rebecca Parker and Rita Nakashima Brock, *Proverbs of Ashes: Violence, Redemptive Suffering, and the Search for What Saves Us* (Boston: Beacon Press, 2001), ch.1.

140. Jane Miller, [pseudo], conversation with the author, New Haven, Connecticut, July 7, 2003.

141. See Nell Painter's discussion of slavery and religion in *Soul Murder and Slavery*, 22–23.

142. Alexander McFarlane and Bessel van der Kolk, "Trauma and Its Challenge to Society," in *Traumatic Stress*, 25.

143. "McFarlane and van der Kolk, "Trauma and Its Challenge to Society," 56.

144. "Selving Faith," *Religion, Scholarship, and Higher Eduction*, ed. by Andrea Sterk (Notre Dame: University of Notre Dame Press, 2002), 145.

145. See Judith Butler, "Contingent Foundations," *Feminist Contentions: A Philosophical Exchange*, ed. Seyla Benhabib et.al. (New York: Routledge, 1995), 46.

146. For a detailed assessment of the possibilities and limitations of poststructuralism in relation to trauma survivors, see Jennifer Beste, *God and the Victim*, chapter four.

147. See Serene Jones, "Selving Faith," 144.

148. Serene Jones, "Selving Faith," 145.

149. See Jane Flax, "Thinking Fragments: Psychoanalysis, Feminism, and Postmodernism in the Contemporary West" (Berkeley: The University of California Press, 1990), 218–19, and Susan Brison, *Aftermath*, 104.

3

Healing the Traumatized Self: Theoretical Perspectives

A couple of years ago I taught a class on trauma to undergraduates at a small, liberal arts college. Toward the beginning of the semester, after reading a particularly intense text on trauma, a few students expressed concern about the psychological impact of studying such weighty material. They observed that learning about trauma is "important," since it is a reality that affects so many people; at the same time, the study of trauma is "depressing," since it can make one feel the burden of what others have endured. In essence, the students were pointing to what some trauma theorists call "indirect" trauma—the sense of despair and despondence that can become instilled in those who learn about others' traumatic experiences. After their initial foray into the study of trauma, the students were wondering: Is there hope in the aftermath of traumatic violence? Are survivors doomed to remain caught in the cycles of trauma that mark their lives—the patterns of dissociation, intrusive memories, hyperarousal? Or are there ways to break these cycles and begin anew?

Trauma theorists answer this last question with a resounding "yes," and the concerns raised by my students indicate that an elaboration of this "yes" is crucial to any discussion of trauma. When trauma theorists describe the extent of the damage trauma can cause, they paint a picture that sounds bleak indeed. It is sometimes hard to imagine that people can recover from such extensive harm, but in fact many do; and so trauma theorists also analyze their multiple paths of recovery, giving us insight into the sources of human resilience as well as a more balanced, accurate view of the dynamics of trauma. In exploring how recovery occurs, trauma theorists thus temper their otherwise sobering discussion with a note of hope—a note which communicates the basic truth that trauma need not have the final word. As the comments of my students indicate, this note is one that many people find helpful to hear.

While it is crucial to explore the recovery process, such exploration must proceed with caution. Those who study trauma indicate that although people often show remarkable resourcefulness and resilience, not all traumatized people recover. Moreover, recovery takes place to varying degrees and in different ways; and even those who experience it to the fullest are not the same after their traumas as they were before. In fact, some trauma scholars are reluctant even to use the terms "healing" and "recovery," since such terms may seem to imply that the survivor gets his or her "old" self back again. Others use this language, either because they do not see it as problematic or because they lack better alternatives. Even those who are comfortable with the language of healing or recovery, though, stress that healing does not mean that survivors go back to "normal," as though nothing ever happened. Trauma leaves a mark that cannot be erased. But survivors can reach a point where the trauma no longer seems so overwhelming—a point where, as one friend put it, "you finally find that things just don't seem so bad anymore."

In this chapter I examine what enables some survivors to arrive at this place where things don't seem so bad—or, where they possibly even seem quite good. I do so by summarizing central insights of trauma scholars about the process of recovery from trauma. In constructing this summary, an unavoidable difficulty surfaces: The descriptions of healing that trauma scholars offer are often somewhat vague. A good reason for this exists, however: Healing from trauma is something of a mystery. It is hard to say why a particular treatment helps one person and not the next, or what exactly made it successful. There exists no comprehensive blueprint for healing, no map that details precisely how one can move from traumatization to health.

Despite this ambiguity, trauma theorists generally agree on two matters related to healing from trauma. First, they understand healing as a reconstitution of the traumatized self. Since trauma fractures the self, healing involves restoring to the self some measure of wholeness or coherence by reintegrating its shattered fragments—for example, the fragments of memory, agency, language, and self-image. Second, trauma theorists suggest that integrating the traumatized self involves several phases or stages of healing. These phases do not represent a neat, linear series of steps that survivors move through in exact sequence; as Herman observes, healing is a messy, complex, and dialectical process.[1] They do, however, provide an organized way to talk about the healing process and illuminate some of its basic principles and goals. Drawing most heavily on Herman's work, I now turn to three central phases of trauma healing. An outline of them provides the theoretical basis for the reconstruction of Christian nonviolence that I begin to develop in the next chapter.

ESTABLISHING SAFETY

Trauma theorists often assert that healing from traumatic violence begins with the vitally important task of establishing safety for trauma survivors. For some survivors, this involves finding physically secure spaces in which they can live and work. This may happen easily for survivors of single traumas who have a strong social support system; however, it proves more difficult for those who experience violence on an ongoing basis. Some survivors who endure repeated traumas remain financially and emotionally dependent on their perpetrators. Others cannot believe that safe spaces exist.[2] Trauma scholars stress that given the numerous challenges survivors face in creating a physically secure space, it is essential for them to have the help of trusted others who can provide emotional support and material assistance, such as loving family members, friends, and support groups.

Once survivors have established a safe environment, they must work to acquire a sense of psychological safety. Trauma theorists indicate that for many traumatized persons, this entails overcoming the feelings of helplessness, fear, and loss of control they experienced during their traumas and in their aftermath. Often, survivors begin to gain a sense of psychological safety as they work with different treatment modalities, including prescription drugs that diminish anxiety and depression, relaxation and stress inoculation techniques, visual imagery, exercise, and participating in social activities.[3] Moreover, Herman contends that some survivors in this initial stage of healing benefit from psychotherapy that concentrates on the fundamental tasks of controlling intrusive symptoms and restoring basic biological functions, such as eating and sleeping. As they begin to identify and stabilize their emotions and biological rhythms through different treatment modalities, the survivor's sense of self-control and competence may increase, making it possible for them to pursue deeper exploration of the issues raised by their traumatic experiences.[4]

Trauma scholars often underscore that in addition to establishing physical and psychological safety, survivors must also develop a sense of social safety, which Bloom specifically defines as feeling secure with people in larger social settings as well as in interpersonal relationships. In her view, survivors can build this sense of security by participating in socially safe environments that maximize their potential for transformation and growth. She cautions, however, that it is difficult to define precisely how human beings can create these socially safe spaces, partly because we do not have many communities or groups that function as role models, enabling us to see precisely what a socially safe space looks like and how it operates.[5]

As Bloom describes them, however, socially safe social environments have several general features. They provide a context in which individuals have the freedom to assume responsibility for their own lives, and in which they are listened to and affirmed. Moreover, socially safe spaces foster relationships marked by mutual cooperation and thoughtfulness, human connections in which people express commitment to the well-being of the group's other members. Some scholars see families as a unit that can provide such a secure setting; in reality, however, they often fail to do so.[6] Given the limitations of family resources, and the ways families often harm rather than support their members, some look to support groups, religious communities, and other collectivities to function as alternative socially safe spaces.

Herman emphasizes that the creation of a physically, psychologically, and socially safe environment often comes with a high cost to trauma survivors. It may require them to take risks, such as venturing to live alone or trusting others. In addition, creating a secure environment sometimes forces survivors to make difficult choices that significantly alter the material character of their lives. For example, some domestic violence survivors must give up their homes, friends, and jobs because extricating themselves from their abusive relationships involves relocating to a new area.[7] For many victims, these costs are simply too daunting. However, others who make such changes find that they begin to repair their self-esteem, sense of competence, and agency. When survivors reclaim their sense of security, they can take charge of their lives and develop a sense of empowerment and conviction—which, in turn, makes it possible to continue with the healing process.

NARRATING THE TRAUMA

Traditional Talk-Based Approaches

When trauma survivors establish safety, they create the conditions that enable them to undertake what trauma scholars often describe as the second phase of healing: coming to terms with the trauma by constructing a trauma narrative. But why does narrating the trauma often make a positive contribution to the survivor's healing process? What is it about telling their stories of trauma that lessens the traumatic symptoms they experience? Are different approaches to creating a trauma narrative any more or less productive? Although trauma theorists acknowledge that the precise relationship between narrative and trauma healing remains unclear, they offer several explanations that help account for how and why narration helps some survivors.

At a most basic level, many trauma theorists contend that narrating the trauma can help survivors heal by enabling them to integrate the event into their personal narratives and thereby gain a sense of wholeness or coherence. Recall that trauma theorists often indicate that part of what gives human beings a sense of wholeness is to be able to gather the multiple stories of their lives into a broader narrative framework that holds together and has meaning. Traumatic events, however, are so overwhelming that they resist integration into this framework; instead, they stand outside of it and call it into question. When survivors narrate their traumas, they resist this disintegration by translating these experiences into language and thereby claiming them as part—albeit a painful part—of their broader life story or history.

Trauma scholars note several ways in which this integration of the trauma into the survivor's life story can help to transform their traumatic symptoms. First, contextualizing the trauma into a broader narrative framework helps survivors begin to overcome their persistent sense of being stuck in the traumatic moment.[8] Recall that trauma survivors often become preoccupied with their traumas, which makes them feel embedded in the past and disconnected from the present. Part of what makes it possible for them to get "unstuck" is to establish a temporal timeline by creating a narrative that locates the trauma in the context of their life story. Repeatedly retelling the trauma story and placing it in the context of "before" and "after" helps the individual to see the trauma not as the one moment that defines their life but as part of a bigger story or ongoing narrative. As the individual retells this story, he or she puts the event into a framework that both recognizes its reality and offers hope for a different future—a future not dominated by the experience of trauma. While this contextualization may not entirely eliminate their traumatic symptoms, it can lessen their intensity and take away their power to retraumatize.

Second, trauma theorists often assert that narrating the trauma enables some survivors to identify and process emotions associated with their traumatic memories. According to Herman, when survivors create trauma narratives, they must move beyond recalling the "facts" of the traumatic experience to discuss their subjective responses—what they feel, see, smell, taste, and hear.[9] Often, survivors express horror at the violence they have endured, and many report feeling anger, despair, shame, and sadness. In addition, some survivors experience profound grief over things they have lost, such as their positive view of themselves, attachment to others, and full range of emotions.[10] Brison observes that while exploring these subjective responses is painful, it can help transform the traumatic character of the memory. By interacting with their traumas in a supportive context, survivors can explore the painful emotions their memories evoke in a setting where they encounter compassion rather than the threat of danger.[11] This takes away some of the isolation invoked by the trauma and enables them to begin to alter their emotions, lessening their pain.

In addition to establishing a temporal timeline and modifying intense emotions, trauma scholars often contend that constructing a trauma narrative can foster healing by allowing survivors to regain a sense of agency and control over intrusive memories. Brison asserts that whereas interpersonal traumas disempower victims by reducing them to an object of their perpetrator's speech or action, narrating the trauma empowers survivors by restoring their voice.[12] In her view, survivors who tell their trauma stories exercise control over the memories that have recurred against their will. They decide how much to disclose and to whom.[13] While this telling itself may be "compulsively repeated" or "out of control," survivors "can control certain aspects of the narrative and that control, repeatedly exercised, leads to greater control over the memories themselves, making them less intrusive and giving them the kind of meaning that enables them to be integrated into the rest of life."[14]

Trauma theorists emphasize that establishing this control does not happen easily. In fact, it usually requires multiple narrations of the trauma story. Herman observes that survivors often alternate between moving closer to the trauma and withdrawing, claiming its reality and then minimizing its impact.[15] Even after multiple tellings survivors may remain uncertain about the "facts" of the trauma and its meaning for their lives. Due to the trauma's unresolved nature, they may continue to carry its effects in their bodies, spirits, and minds; however, these symptoms often lessen progressively as victims continue to discuss their traumas. At the end of each telling, they may experience the story as "over and complete"—at least for the time being.[16] This sense of completion becomes more permanent as new details and insight on the trauma emerge. When a fuller account develops, the survivor gains a sense that the event had a beginning and end, a circumscribed location in space and time.[17]

While many trauma theorists emphasize the power of creating a trauma narrative to restore the survivor's sense of control and coherence, Brison also cautions that the act of narration can impede recovery, if it binds the survivor to one unchanging account of the past (such as when she needs to have her story "right" for the purposes of a trial). In her view, survivors must ultimately engage in

> telling to live, which I now see as a kind of letting go, playing with the past in order not to be held back as one springs away from it. After gaining enough control over the story to be able to tell it, perhaps one has to give it up, in order to retell it, without having to "get it right," without fear of betraying it, to be able to rewrite the past in different ways, leading up to an infinite variety of unforeseeable futures.[18]

Here, Brison suggests that narrating the trauma facilitates healing not by giving the survivor a sense that the future is predictable and the course of her life is completely within her control (which it is not), but rather by making it possible for her to carry on with courage and confidence in the midst of an uncertain world.[19]

Despite the differing views that trauma scholars hold about how narrative helps survivors, then, they generally agree that the creation of a trauma narrative is an integral part of healing for many traumatized persons. They also, however, stress that survivors often run into difficulties when constructing this narrative. One common problem is dissociation: In some instances, survivors cannot talk about their traumas because they cannot remember the details surrounding these events or even whole periods of time. Trauma scholars observe that when this happens, clinicians may use a variety of techniques to help survivors uncover their dissociated memories, including hypnosis, individual or group therapy, art, and dance/movement therapy.[20] Herman asserts that the easiest way to recall traumatic memories is to explore memories the survivor has: "As the patient experiences the full emotional impact of facts she already knows, new recollections usually emerge spontaneously."[21] In her view, many survivors find that thinking about their responses to nontraumatic events, exploring the meaning of their physical sensations, and discussing their past and present relationships help them uncover dissociated, traumatic memories.[22]

Some trauma theorists contend that a cognitive-behavioral therapy called "imaginal exposure therapy" also can unlock and transform traumatic memories. According to Barbara Rothbaum and Edna Foa, imaginal exposure is based on the belief that "short-term suffering will lead to long-term benefit."[23] More specifically, they explain that those who use this therapy find that for some survivors, confronting the trauma in a state of relaxation can foster healing. Imaginal exposure sessions thus begin with relaxation exercises; the survivor then recalls and interacts with their trauma. For example, they may imagine being back in the trauma and recount the incident as if it were happening again. Or, they may write an account of the trauma and read it aloud. Rothbaum and Foa report that while the survivor's first exposure to the trauma often produces a narrative with few details, subsequent sessions aim to generate a more complete description by exploring the emotional and physiological reactions that the traumatic memory generates.[24] After the exposure and analysis of their response, survivors again work on relaxation. By confronting their trauma in a controlled setting in which they take charge of the remembering, survivors can modify their fear and begin to transform the traumatic structure of the memory.[25]

Herman describes a similar treatment called "direct exposure."[26] Like imaginal exposure, this approach is based on the conviction that controlled reliving can help the survivor overcome the terror associated with their trauma. In direct exposure, survivors confront, for a limited period of time and in a safe setting, images or symbols related to (but different from) their traumas. For example, a war veteran may listen to the sound of a helicopter or watch a movie about combat.[27]

What makes this exposure to the trauma a potential source of healing, a way to unlock and transform traumatic memories? One theory holds that part of what makes it possible for survivors to narrate their traumas is to see these experiences symbolized in ways both similar to and different from their own stories. The similarity between the images and the survivor's experience activates the traumatic memory and enables them to interact with it; the difference allows the traumatic structure of the memory to be transformed.[28] According to van der Kolk and his colleagues, the most critical difference in modifying traumatic memories is the context in which the survivors engage the images of their traumas. When traumatized individuals interact with these images in a secure setting, they encounter them in a place where they have assistance in monitoring and processing the emotions they evoke. Here, they can begin to regain a sense of control and develop confidence that even though remembering the traumatic event proves difficult, they have the strength and support necessary to do this and to deal with the pain it causes.[29]

Narration, however, does not work for everyone. Trauma scholars report that in addition to having dissociated memories, survivors often face other obstacles that make it a difficult task. Some find that their inability to feel emotions leaves them without motivation to create an ongoing narrative.[30] Others experience a loss of self and voice that causes them to doubt their own memories.[31] Still others lack the social support needed to recall and discuss their traumas.[32] Finally, in some instances, survivors can recall the facts of their traumas but find it too risky or painful to verbally communicate about these experiences. Years of secrecy and silence around their traumas condition some victims to fear disclosure about their inner lives and emotions. Past experiences of rejection, criticism, or abandonment render them unable to trust their listeners enough to talk about their traumas.[33]

Survivors of repeated traumas may face an especially hard task when it comes to this stage of trauma recovery, partly because their defense mechanisms are more likely to be deeply entrenched and thus more difficult to unlearn. In addition, placing one's traumas in a broader narrative framework will more likely promote healing when that framework contains multiple stories of health and happiness, rather than multiple stories of trauma. Those who have endured repeated traumas that began when they were young may lack the positive experiences that enable them to contextualize their traumas in a framework that includes a vision of a future in which they flourish. Put differently, the central goal of narrating the trauma—contextualizing it in a larger framework of memory and meaning—is to reintegrate the self, restoring its coherence or wholeness; but some survivors may never have established a coherent self that they can later "put back together again."

Nonverbal Approaches

Trauma scholars often argue that even when survivors do not find success with the traditional "talking cure," healing is still possible. Traumatized persons who cannot integrate their traumatic experiences through verbal narration may turn to nonverbal approaches as a means to "narrate" or tell their stories. Often done in conjunction with talking therapies, nonverbal approaches involve intentionally using, within a therapeutic context, art or creative activities such as painting, drama, or dance.[34] They are based on the premise that one can speak through nonverbal as well as verbal forms. As Bonnie Meekums puts it, "a gesture can express feeling; a painting, drama or poem can tell a story; and the structuring of space can say much about the person's relationships."[35] For many survivors, the use of creative modalities provides a fruitful way to connect with their inner selves and communicate about their traumas. Survivors can tell their stories through their bodies, rather than in words. Once externalized through the body this story can, in some instances, be translated with the help of others into a coherent verbal narrative.[36]

David Read Johnson observes that while professionals who work with survivors employ approaches that involve a diversity of art modalities, some common elements characterize sessions that focus on nonverbal expression.[37] He explains that usually, a typical session begins with a discussion about how the client is doing and what issues they want to address. Instead of exploring these issues through verbal conversation, the therapist and client use an art medium as a way to communicate about the problem. They may begin with warmup exercises that enable the client to relax, such as drawing or scribbling on paper (for art therapy), stretching or jogging (for dance/movement therapy), or making noises on a musical instrument (for music therapy). Once they complete the introductory exercises, the therapist and client delve more deeply into the art medium. The therapist may ask the client to design whatever she chooses, or give her a specific task, such as to draw a picture of her parents or feelings of sadness. The client and therapist may then reflect on the meaning of what she has created. In some instances, the therapist leaves it up to the individual to explore the artwork's significance. In other situations, therapists offer their own ideas about what the art might mean in the larger context of the client's life.[38]

Johnson further explains how nonverbal treatments promote healing from trauma by noting an important difference between nonverbal therapy work and artistic training. Whereas artistic training involves a structured, disciplined process of modeling basic forms, nonverbal therapies involve unstructured or loosely structured creative activities that take place in a relaxed atmosphere. Johnson observes that this "play" setting enables clients to explore, grow, and have fun. They may "let go" enough to move beyond intellectualization and connect with their internal worlds, which, in turn, makes it possible to express thoughts and feelings they could not communicate in words.[39] According to Charles Schaefer, creative acts emerge partly from the unconscious and thus can reveal images and memories buried in survivors' bodies and minds. This is why abused children often express thoughts and feelings they are not consciously aware of through drawings or in puppet play.[40]

One theory holds that the "play" which characterizes nonverbal modalities can help survivors unearth and express traumatic memories partly because of its emphasis on the body. Many trauma theorists believe that since trauma is stored in the body, physical experiences can unlock dissociated traumatic memories and help survivors confront hidden dimensions of their traumas. For example, Letty Mills and Judith Daniluk describe one study that examined the experiences of five trauma survivors who turned to dance therapy.[41] For these survivors, dance movement provided a way to get "'out of their heads,'" so that they could connect with and express previously unknown or denied aspects of their selves.[42] As one woman says, "I knew somehow my body would tell me the truth . . . the surprise was how deeply my body felt the things that happened to me . . . for the first time I understood what body memory means."[43] Similarly, Patricia Weaver Francisco, a rape survivor, describes how she turned to "body work" after having little success integrating her trauma through traditional talk-based therapies. In working with a specialist who helped her to "read" and analyze her body's voice by identifying and interpreting its sensations, Weaver was able to access the feelings and ideas behind these sensations.[44]

One advantage to nonverbal approaches is that they can help survivors express their feelings without becoming overwhelmed. Speaking through art forms can give one psychological distance from one's traumas. As one individual explains,

> I was sort of talking about the drawing. It was easier because I had something here to hold up. It was almost like having a mask in front of me, it was almost like something with me, as if I was hiding behind a mask really and it was the painting that was speaking . . . It's not me speaking it's the dance speaking. It's not me speaking it's the drama speaking. . . .[45]

Nonverbal treatments can thus facilitate the communication of survivors' stories while providing them with some protection against becoming flooded with affect.

This does not mean, however, that nonverbal modalities are necessarily accompanied by little emotion. At times, such approaches evoke intense feelings. For example, the participants in the dance therapy study that Mills and Daniluk describe found that particular movements or music evoked flashbacks of their traumatic experiences. The authors report that though difficult, re-experiencing these traumatic memories provided them with a chance to explore symptoms that needed to be addressed. Some elected to process these memories by talking about them; others did not. Given their traumatic past, the survivors found it empowering to have the freedom to choose silence. They discovered that not having to talk helped them avoid "'spoiling' a significant moment of bodily connection."[46]

In addition to helping survivors uncover and express traumatic memories, nonverbal approaches can help them overcome their sense of alienation from their bodies. Recall that traumatized persons often experience a split between their bodies and minds that stems from dissociative defenses learned during the traumas and in their aftermath. As one individual remarked, "I had spent most of my life feeling that my body either walked in front of me or behind me. . . ."[47] Mills and Daniluk note that for participants in the study on dance therapy, both synchronized and spontaneous movement facilitated reconnection with their bodies by making them more aware of specific body parts.[48] By reuniting with their bodies, they became more attuned to and comfortable with their physical and emotional sensations. This enabled them to respect their bodies, motivating them to give more attention to self-care. As a result of these changes, they regained a sense of wholeness and integration that their traumas had destroyed.[49]

For some survivors, nonverbal modalities not only facilitate reconnection with their memories and bodies, but also enable them to create and embody new, positive possibilities. For example, drama therapists Craig Haen and Kenneth Brannon found that performing roles helps some survivors to internalize the positive values of the roles they play. In working with traumatized boys in one long-term care facility, they discovered that the boys played out three roles time and again: superheroes, monsters, and babies.[50] Many who acted out the superhero roles chose this part because the superheroes, like themselves, had a traumatic past. But unlike the children, they had overcome this adversity and gone on to lead successful lives. By flourishing despite their difficult times, the superheroes gave the boys hope that they could do the same. As they reflected on the positive aspects of the roles, the boys accessed their own inner strengths. One eight-year-old remarked, "I store all of my characters in my heart. Whenever I need one, I pull it out and it helps me."[51]

Those who study nonverbal modalities often emphasize that while some traumatized persons make progress in healing through nonverbal treatments, these approaches do not work for all survivors. Some are inhibited by their belief that they have no artistic talent.[52] Others remain unable to access their creative abilities due to their damaged trust in themselves and other people.[53] In addition, many survivors, particularly those who have suffered sexual abuse, feel uncomfortable with their bodies and thus shy away from treatment approaches that focus on the body as a means of expression. Still others fear any treatment that attempts to disclose their innermost thoughts and feelings. As Meekums observes, for an individual who "has learned to survive by hiding the self in any number of ways, such revelation could be experienced as threatening."[54] Given the risks of nonverbal treatments, Susan Simonds stresses that those who use them must make sure survivors prepare for their work with these approaches. They can do this by identifying what might help them feel secure in the midst of remembering, discussing their expectations of what will happen if they recall past traumas, and talking about their anticipated responses.[55]

Many trauma scholars conclude, however, that when undertaken with care, nonverbal modalities can play a significant role in the survivor's healing process. They can help bring hidden aspects of the self into conscious awareness and integrate traumatic memories into the survivor's personal narrative. In addition, nonverbal therapies can enable survivors to internalize new, positive values and behaviors. As Herman notes,

> The major work of the second stage is accomplished . . . when the patient reclaims her own history and feels renewed hope and energy for engagement with life. Time starts to move again. When the "action of telling a story" has come to its conclusion, the traumatic experience truly belongs to the past.[56]

To say that the trauma belongs to the past does not mean that survivors forget their traumas or leave them entirely behind. At this stage of the healing process, survivors still carry their traumas with them but do so in a new way.[57] Incorporated into their personal narrative, the trauma loses its power to retraumatize.[58] When this happens, survivors cease to feel stuck in the past. Their myopic vision has expanded so that they no longer remain fixated on their traumatic experiences, and these experiences thus no longer exclusively define their identities, their sense of who they are.

RETEMPORALIZATION

Trauma scholars indicate that survivors who have placed their traumas in the larger context of their lives as events in the past can focus on a final task of healing: their "retemporalization."[59] Once survivors have temporally located their traumas by contextualizing them in a broader narrative framework, they can themselves experience a different orientation toward time. No longer consumed by the past, they can fully immerse themselves in the present by deepening their friendships, developing concrete plans for their future, and putting these plans into action. In short, they can continue to develop their "new" self as they move into the world, fully engaged with the present and empowered by a hopeful vision for what is to come.

Herman asserts that for some survivors, this reconnection with the present requires shedding parts of their "old" selves that their traumas imposed. In her view, survivors may need to continue working to let go of their fear of intimacy, guilt, depression, or anxiety.[60] As they move deeper into the recovery process and become more actively engaged in rebuilding their lives, survivors often find that it gets easier to relinquish or forgive parts of their traumatized selves. As one abuse survivor remarked about her career as a pornographic movie star,

> I'm not so hard on myself these days. Maybe it's because I'm so busy taking care of a three-year-old son, a husband, a house, and two cats. I look back at [my former self] and I understand her; I know why she did what she did. It was because she felt it was better to live than to die.[61]

Herman asserts that as they let go of parts of their traumatized selves, survivors may hold on to positive qualities or behaviors that resulted from the trauma, "even while recognizing that any gain was achieved at far too great a price."[62]

For some survivors, developing their new self also involves disclosing their traumas to others. While many survivors in the second stage of healing narrate their traumas to a therapist or trusted friend, they may in the third stage reveal their traumatic past to others as well.[63] At this point, survivors often find that disclosing past traumas builds intimacy in relationships and serves as a source of inspiration for others.[64] While many prefer to tell their story only to friends and select family members, others talk about their experiences publicly. Some even confront their perpetrators or bystanders who refused to help them. Herman notes that such confrontations can be quite difficult for survivors, since offenders sometimes respond with denial or anger. However, if the truth-telling is well-planned the disclosure may empower the survivor, even if those confronted respond negatively.[65] Speaking the truth enables some survivors to feel they have overcome their fears of their perpetrators and freed themselves from the dynamics of harmful relationships.[66]

Trauma scholars note that many survivors find that support groups provide a helpful context in which to disclose their traumas and build life-giving relationships. Herman, for instance, contends that while early in the healing process support groups focus on establishing physical, psychological, and social safety, they can later provide a setting in which survivors explore the meaning of their traumas. Many victims find it empowering to share their stories in a group and hear the stories of others; knowing that others have had similar experiences can help them overcome the isolation that their traumas imposed.[67] Some survivors also find that support groups make it possible for them to reconnect with aspects of their former selves that their traumas had buried. For example, Brison asserts that groups can enable survivors to develop compassion for their traumatized selves by empathizing with others. In hearing the stories of others who survived traumas similar to their own, victims realize that these others are not to blame for their traumas and thus stop blaming themselves.[68]

In addition to shedding aspects of their "old" selves and developing new relationships, trauma theorists argue that constructing a hopeful vision of the future represents another integral dimension of retemporalization. Recall that some survivors have a foreshortened sense of the future. Consumed by intrusive post-traumatic symptoms that generate sadness, fear, and despair, they remain unable to imagine a future that is different from their traumatic past. However, once survivors have given their traumas definite temporal and spatial location and thereby gained control over their traumatic symptoms, they can anticipate the future with hope, setting goals for their lives and a plan for how to attain them. For some survivors, this entails returning to aspirations they held prior to their traumas. For others, it involves pursuing new goals and interests. Herman observes that many people at this stage find it helpful to have a "survivor mission,"[69] such as participating in social action, engaging in intellectual pursuits, or reaching out to troubled individuals.[70] Such a mission gives them a sense that their lives have meaning and purpose, for they have now not only transformed their own injuries but also made a contribution to the world that transcends their particular location in space and time.

While survivors at this point have come a long way in the healing process, they may occasionally revisit issues from the earlier phases of healing.[71] For example, in phase three survivors may return to the issue of safety and increase their sense of security by confronting and overcoming specific fears. Brison, for example, lobbied her employers to put a lock on a door in an isolated passageway and install a light in a parking lot where she left her car at night.[72] Other survivors increase their sense of safety by engaging in physical activities that help them overcome insecurities and foster healthy connection with others. They may take part in self-defense classes or go on outings (wilderness trips, camping) in which they rehearse confrontation with danger in a way that builds self-confidence and a sense of control.[73] Herman asserts that through such activities, survivors continue to decondition their stress response to neutral environmental stimuli. In so doing, they restructure their "physiological and psychological responses to fear."[74]

MEANING-MAKING AND HEALING

One key part of the healing process that trauma scholars identify as integral to all three phases is the difficult task of meaning-making. Recall that as meaning-making creatures, human beings often struggle to tell their stories in ways that give themselves a broader sense of purpose for their lives and the world. For trauma survivors, this search for meaning often does not lead them to see the traumas as good or meaningful, but it does allow them to discover that some good has come *after* the trauma, from the recovery process.[75] The specific ways in which survivors arrive at this realization, however, differ from one person to the next.

Trauma theorists name at least four common ways that trauma survivors often find meaning in the aftermath of their traumatic experiences. First, many survivors consider the lessons they have learned about life during their healing process.[76] For example, they discover that after their traumas they no longer take forgranted gifts such as friendship, family, or the beauty of nature. This, in turn, frees them to enjoy life more fully and reorder their priorities so that they spend less time on unimportant matters such as household chores, and more time on cherished ones such as enjoying the companionship of family and friends.[77]

Second, some survivors find meaning after their traumas by focusing on lessons they have learned about themselves. For instance, many find that they have become more compassionate and caring.[78] Others feel psychologically stronger or more confident now that they have endured the difficult times. Despite their clear sense that the world is dangerous and random, they feel internally more secure and believe they can overcome the challenges they face. As one rape survivor put it, "I feel much stronger now, even though I feel vulnerable to being raped in this culture. Part of that rape was to dominate and humiliate me and he didn't succeed at that. I came through with my integrity—I got through those months of hell. The world is more dangerous to me now, but I am . . . stronger, able to handle anything. . . ."[79]

Third, Janoff-Bulman asserts that some survivors find meaning after their traumas by focusing on the benefits they can offer to others.[80] Survivors may use the wisdom and knowledge they have acquired to help people by being an authentic listener to them, by participating in social and political activities that benefit causes related to their traumas, or by taking part in outreach projects that increase public awareness about traumas such as domestic and sexual violence. For many individuals, engaging in such activities affirms that their lives have value and purpose. As one survivor put it, "I feel like everything I've been through adds to what I'm able to offer to other people. That's a great feeling—that's kind of like the spiritual piece of healing. When you feel like somehow it's redeemed and it wasn't all for nothing."[81]

Fourth, some survivors turn to the explicit dimensions of religious faith to help them address questions of meaning. For example, after horrifying experiences some people derive comfort and guidance from their religious beliefs.[82] Others find solace in the notion that God loves them and remains present with them throughout the ups and downs of their lives. One survivor states the matter this way:

> Adversity matures your faith. And my faith and prayers helped me through the whole thing—coping with it I mean. I know God was with me. I've been able to turn it into a stepping stone. You know, I've learned from it and I've grown. And if I can do something to help other people then that makes the whole thing less horrible.[83]

For some survivors, religion has resources to help them integrate what they have learned from their traumas about the fragility of life and the randomness of the world into their overarching view of reality. It offers a cognitive schema through which they can regain a sense of meaning and purpose in light of their traumatic experiences.[84]

While some trauma survivors find solace in specific religious beliefs or doctrines, others turn to religious rituals to help them make meaning. Rituals provide structure and reliability that counters the chaos and randomness of trauma. As one survivor says, "In the church it was the ritual I really liked. Not necessarily all the words because they are very patriarchal and I really got some bad vibes about God the Father. But to just be able to go and sit and relax and know what's going on and have the ritual and worship happen . . . I think there's a real safety in that."[85]

In addition to offering this structure and predictability, rituals create a way for survivors to place their losses within a larger framework. Through ritual, trauma survivors establish connections not only with the divine and their present community but also with the past and the suffering of others. For example, many Christian communities perform the "Prayers of the People" during their Sunday morning worship, in which the congregation prays not only for the healing of their members' own suffering but also for those who suffer around the world. By making this prayer an integral part of their weekly service, churches establish a bonding among people across space and time. This bonding can take away some of the survivors' isolation and give their lives a sense of coherence and continuity.[86]

Some trauma theorists suggest that rituals may also facilitate meaning-making by providing a way to explore deeper aspects of the self that words cannot access. Janine Roberts, for instance, observes that rituals use symbols, and symbols can evoke memories and feelings. More specifically, the embodied and active nature of rituals makes them well-suited to get in touch with emotions and inner worlds.[87] According to Roberts, since rituals "often call on known symbols and action, they offer continuity that can create a sense of safety and facilitate movement into the unknown."[88] While this connection may be painful for some survivors, it can give them a chance to interact with their experiences in a different way and in a new context. One survivor asserts that she has found religious ritual helpful precisely because it "short circuits all that mental trying to think it through. That's always been true for me about ritual—that it just meets some deeper place than reading books or thinking about the trauma or talking about it can. I think that's the power of it."[89] By tapping into this "deeper place," religious ritual gives survivors a chance to experience meaningful connections with others, the divine, and themselves.

This diversity of methods that trauma survivors employ to find meaning in the aftermath of their traumas shares one common element: They all involve connecting the survivor's personal narratives to an overarching narrative that includes larger stories about human life. More specifically, meaning-making after trauma entails linking the individual's story with broader narratives about the divine, other trauma survivors, and human communities. When survivors make such connections, they can mitigate their isolation and begin to see themselves as agents who are part of a struggle for peace and justice that transcends the boundaries of their own lives.

THE DIFFICULT MATTER OF FORGIVENESS

Trauma theorists note that as survivors reconstruct themselves by reconnecting with themselves, others, and the world, they often confront one additional issue: the difficult matter of forgiveness. Should survivors forgive their perpetrators, and if so, under what conditions? Trauma scholars offer differing viewpoints on this matter, partly because the term forgiveness means different things to different people. On the one hand, some consider the language of forgiveness problematic because, in their view, forgiveness—especially when granted before justice has been made—constitutes "cheap grace," which fails to hold the perpetrators accountable for their actions.[90] From this perspective, forgiveness excuses the perpetrator's behavior, which, in turn, grants him or her license to offend again.

Others believe forgiveness is problematic for a different reason: It imposes yet another burden on the survivor. Herman, for instance, argues that the quest to forgive often becomes a "cruel torture," as it remains an inachievable goal for the victim.[91] When one has experienced violent harm at the hands of another human being, forgiveness sometimes is simply too difficult. In Herman's view, forgiveness becomes a more realistic goal when perpetrators admit their wrongdoing, seek repentance, and try to make amends.[92] Marie Fortune, however, notes that most perpetrators never do this. Thus, she argues that the survivor's wider community must take responsibility for repentance and restitution. The church, the legal system, and close family and friends can name the wrong and make justice for victims.[93]

On the other hand, many trauma scholars assert that forgiveness can constitute an important part of the survivor's healing, even when the perpetrators do not repent and reconciliation with them is neither possible nor desirable. Those who argue this point often understand forgiveness not as forgetting or excusing the trauma but as recognizing the wrongdoing and not allowing it to destroy the survivor's spirit.[94] Thus, when survivors forgive their perpetrators they call attention to the fact that what happened was wrong (for otherwise there would be nothing to forgive). At the same time, they let go of their bitterness over the event and thereby refuse to let the perpetrator continue to have significant influence over their lives. As one survivor remarked, "When you forgive someone you give up those feelings that you were holding onto for a long time. And it may have been something you obsessed about and hard to walk away from. But I don't want my perpetrator in my life . . . I want to have a life separate from him. So I want to forgive him and walk away."[95]

Despite their differing views of forgiveness, trauma theorists generally agree that it is extremely difficult. Forgiveness involves recognizing the brokenness of the perpetrators, acknowledging that the harms they commit may stem from their own experiences of violence and injustice. Humanizing one's perpetrator in this way is something survivors can do only when they have healed enough to relate to the world out of their wholeness rather than their brokenness.[96] Thus, some trauma theorists contend that forgiveness should mark the last step in the healing process—if, indeed, the survivor chooses to grant it at all.[97]

Trauma theorists are often careful to balance their discussions of forgiveness with the observation that anger can have a positive force in the survivor's life as well.[98] Understandably, traumatized persons may become angry when they lose their sense of safety, when others lack understanding, or when their perpetrators refuse to show remorse. As Debra Alexander observes, although survivors may express this anger in destructive ways, it often has healthy dimensions that enable it to function as a healing force in their lives.[99] For example, anger can inspire individuals to take action that initiates social change. It can also build and reinforce a positive self-concept by reminding survivors that the violence done to them was wrong and that they deserve better treatment. Like forgiveness, then, anger draws on the survivor's own power to make a positive contribution to the reconstruction of the self.

Unfortunately, those around survivors often discourage them from feeling and expressing anger, either by minimizing the trauma or by appealing to beliefs about love and forgiveness. This attempt to suppress anger and only show forgiveness fails to recognize the ways each of these responses, when left unchecked by the other, may prove problematic. Anger without forgiveness can result in actions that continue cycles of violence, and forgiveness without recognizing one's anger and demanding justice can lead to "cheap grace." Thus, these responses are not incompatible but rather two that can, in some instances, work together to help survivors reconstruct their self-concept, agency, and human relationships.

TRAUMA HEALING AND COMMUNITIES

In trauma scholars' descriptions of healing, the importance of healthy connections with others stands out as a central theme that undergirds each phase. Recall that in discussing the first phase of healing, trauma theorists stress that loving friends and family members can play a crucial role in helping survivors establish a safe environment. Similarly, in describing the second, they emphasize that survivors will more likely construct a trauma narrative when empathic others hear the story and respond with compassion. Finally, when talking about the third phase of healing, trauma theorists underscore that an integral part is developing and deepening healthy relationships. In all these ways and more, healing requires the constant presence of others and a strong social support system. Some traumatized persons find such support in a relationship with a trusted individual, but communities also can provide crucial assistance to survivors during the healing process. Families, support groups, religious organizations, and other social groups can offer financial, emotional, and spiritual help that survivors need to integrate their traumas and rebuild their lives.

In the following pages, I want to focus on the particular contributions to recovery that religious communities can make. Many resources that trauma theorists identify as integral to healing—narratives, rituals, caring listeners—are resources these communities have. Religious communities have their own narratives, perform rituals, and, at least when they function well, bring together people who care for each other and listen to each other's stories. While each religious tradition has its own distinctive resources, I concentrate on those of the Christian tradition. How might Christianity's narratives and practices foster the healing of traumatized persons? If traumatic violence can become internal to socially constructed people and the communities they form, then how can Christian communities, which are themselves constructed as sites of violence, help to transform this violence?

These questions are important to explore. Although the church has sanctioned violence in many ways, it also has provided innumerable people with support and care in times of crisis. As we saw in chapter 2, some individuals do discover in these communities sources of support (even as others do not). Examining some of the potential resources these communities have to offer illuminates why this may be the case. In addition, it points to ways that Christian communities might more effectively address the reality of trauma with which many of their members contend.

Each of the next three chapters explores specific resources of Christian communities by theologically reflecting on a phase of trauma recovery: establishing safety, narrating the trauma, and retemporalization. In developing these theological reflections, I consider both how the experiences of trauma survivors may challenge traditional Christian beliefs and practices and how Christian communities, despite their participation in the brokenness of the world, may nonetheless address the needs of traumatized persons. Ultimately, this analysis facilitates my larger theoretical goal: reconceptualizing Christian nonviolence to include not only resisting external violence but also transforming internalized, traumatic violence.

NOTES

1. Herman, *Trauma and Recovery*, 155.
2. Susan L. Simonds, *Bridging the Silence: Nonverbal Modalities in the Treatment of Adult Survivors of Childhood Sexual Abuse* (New York: W. W. Norton & Company, Inc., 1994), 80.
3. Van der Kolk, McFarlane, and van der Hart, "A General Approach to Treatment," 426; Jon G. Allen, *Coping with Trauma*, 279–288.
4. Herman, *Trauma and Recovery*, 161–74.
5. Bloom, *Creating Sanctuary*, 117.
6. Bloom, *Creating Sanctuary*, 118.
7. See Herman, *Trauma and Recovery*, 172.
8. See Dori Laub, "Bearing Witness."
9. Herman, *Trauma and Recovery*, 177–79.
10. Herman, *Trauma and Recovery*, 188–95.
11. Van der Kolk, McFarlane, and van der Hart, "A General Approach to Treatment," 430–31.
12. Brison, *Aftermath*, 68.
13. Brison, *Aftermath*, 54.
14. Brison, *Aftermath*, 54.
15. *Trauma and Recovery*, 177.
16. Aaron Mishara, "Narrative and Psychotherapy—The Phenomenology of Healing," *American Journal of Psychotherapy*, 49, no. 2 (Spring 1995): 81–90.
17. Laub, "Bearing Witness," 69.
18. Brison, *Aftermath*, 103.
19. Brison, *Aftermath*, 104.
20. See van der Kolk, *Psychological Trauma* (Washington, DC: American Psychiatric Publishing, 1987); Herman, *Trauma and Recovery*, 185–87; and David Read Johnson, *Essays on the Creative Arts Therapies: Imaging the Birth of a Profession* (Springfield, IL: Charles C Thomas Publisher, 1999).
21. Herman, *Trauma and Recovery*, 184.
22. Herman, *Trauma and Recovery*, chapter 7.
23. Rothbaum and Foa, "Cognitive-Behavioral Therapy for PTSD," in *Traumatic Stress*, 503.

24. Rothbaum and Foa, "Cognitive-Behavioral Therapy for PTSD," 504.
25. Rothbaum and Foa, "Cognitive-Behavioral Therapy for PTSD," 492.
26. Herman, *Trauma and Recovery*, 181.
27. Susannah Mozley, personal conversation with the author.
28. Van der Kolk, McFarlane, and van der Hart, "A General Approach to Treatment," 430.
29. Van der Kolk, McFarlane, and van der Hart, "A General Approach to Treatment," 430.
30. Brison, *Aftermath*, 50.
31. Susan L. Simonds, *Bridging the Silence*, 3.
32. Brison, *Aftermath*, 62.
33. Simonds, *Bridging the Silence*, 2.
34. Bonnie Meekums, *Creative Group Therapy for Women Survivors of Child Sexual Abuse* (London: Jessica Kingsley Publishers, 2000), 47.
35. Meekums, *Creative Group Therapy*, 57. See also Maralynn M. Hagood, *The Use of Art in Counseling Child and Adult Survivors of Sexual Abuse* (London: Jessica Kingsley Publishers, 2000).
36. Simonds, *Bridging the Silence*, 4.
37. David Read Johnson, *Essays on the Creative Arts Therapies*, 124–25.
38. Johnson, *Essays on the Creative Arts Therapies*, 124–25.
39. Johnson, *Essays on the Creative Arts Therapies*, 25.
40. Charles Schaefer also notes that children can, through play, enact conscious thoughts and feelings as well. The communication process in play thus can take place on two levels, the conscious and the unconscious. "What Is Play and Why Is It Therapeutic?" *The Therapeutic Powers of Play* (Northvale, NJ: Jason Aronson, Inc., 1993), 6–7.
41. Mills and Daniluka, "Her Body Speaks: The Experience of Dance Therapy for Women Survivors of Child Sexual Abuse," *Journal of Counseling and Development* 80:1 (Winter 2002): 77–85.
42. Mills and Daniluka, "Her Body Speaks," 83.
43. Mills and Daniluka, "Her Body Speaks," 80.
44. Patricia Weaver Francisco, *Telling: A Memoir of Rape and Recovery* (New York: Cliff Street Books, 1999), 148.
45. Qtd. in Meekums, *Creative Group Therapy*, 97.
46. Mills and Daniluka, "Her Body Speaks," 82.
47. Qtd. in Mills and Daniluk, "Her Body Speaks," 79.
48. Mills and Daniluka, "Her Body Speaks," 80.
49. Mills and Daniluka, "Her Body Speaks," 80.
50. Craig Haen and Kenneth H. Brannon, "Superheroes, Monsters, and Babies: Roles of Strength, Destruction, and Vulnerability for Emotionally Disturbed Boys," *The Arts in Psychotherapy* 29 (2002): 31–40.
51. Haen and Brannon, "Superheroes, Monsters, and Babies," 39.
52. Meekums, *Creative Group Therapy*, 99.
53. Meekums, *Creative Group Therapy*, 99.
54. Meekums, *Creative Group Therapy*, 99.
55. Simonds, *Breaking the Silence*, 138–39.
56. Herman, *Trauma and Recovery*, 195.

57. Laub, "An Event Without Witness," 91–92.

58. Laub, "An Event Without Witness," 75–92; Herman, *Trauma and Recovery*, 228.

59. I thank Shannon Craigo-Snell for suggesting this word to capture the essence of the third phase of recovery. Trauma theorists do not use it.

60. Herman, *Trauma and Recovery*, 203.

61. Qtd. in Herman, *Trauma and Recovery*, 204.

62. Herman, *Trauma and Recovery*, 204.

63. Herman, *Trauma and Recovery*, 200–201.

64. Herman, *Trauma and Recovery*, 215–17.

65. By "well-planned," Herman means that the disclosure takes place only when the survivor is ready for it and has adequate support in strategizing, rehearsing, and dealing with the responses of others. See Herman, *Trauma and Recovery*, 200–201.

66. Herman, *Trauma and Recovery*, 201.

67. Herman, *Trauma and Recovery*, 233–36.

68. Brison, *Aftermath*, 63.

69. Herman, *Trauma and Recovery*, 207.

70. Herman, *Trauma and Recovery*, 208.

71. Herman, *Trauma and Recovery*, 197.

72. Brison, *Aftermath*, 61.

73. Herman, *Trauma and Recovery*, 198.

74. Herman, *Trauma and Recovery*, 198.

75. Brison, *Aftermath*, 20.

76. Janoff-Bulman, *Shattered Assumptions*, 135.

77. Janoff-Bulman, *Shattered Assumptions*, 136.

78. Janoff-Bulman, *Shattered Assumptions*, 137.

79. Qtd. in Janoff-Bulman, *Shattered Assumptions*, 137.

80. Janoff-Bulman, *Shattered Assumptions*, 138–39.

81. Kathryn Douglas [pseudo.], interview with the author, Washington, DC, July 16, 2003.

82. Wendy S. Overcash, Lawrence G. Calhoun, Arnie Cann, and Richard G. Tedeschi, "Coping with Crises: An Examination of the Impact of Traumatic Events on Religious Beliefs," *The Journal of Genetic Psychology* 157 (December 1996): 455–64.

83. Qtd. in Wendy S. Overcash, et al., "Coping with Crises," 461.

84. Overcash, et al. "Coping with Crises," 455–64.

85. Sally Morgan [pseudo.], conversation with the author, New Haven, CT, July 8, 2003.

86. See Alexander McFarlane and Bessel A. van der Kolk, "Trauma and Its Challenge to Society," 24–46 and Marten W. deVries, "Trauma in Cultural Perspective," in *Traumatic Stress*, 398–413.

87. See Janine Roberts, "Beyond Words: The Power of Rituals," in *Beyond Talk Therapy: Using Movement and Expressive Techniques in Clinical Therapy*, ed. Daniel J. Wiener (Washington, DC: American Psychological Association, 1999), 55–78.

88. Roberts, "Beyond Words," 57.

89. Kathryn Douglas [pseudo.], conversation with the author, Washington, DC, July 16, 2003.

90. See Marie Fortune, "Forgiveness: The Last Step," in *Violence Against Women and Children*, eds. Carol J. Adams and Marie M. Fortune (New York: Continuum, 1995), 201–6.

91. Herman, *Trauma and Recovery*, 190. Given the space constraints of this chapter, my discussion of forgiveness addresses only the survivors' forgiveness of their perpetrators. For those survivors who struggle with feelings of guilt, however, one could also talk about their forgiveness of themselves.

92. Herman, *Trauma and Recovery*, 190.

93. Fortune, "Forgiveness: The Last Step," 202.

94. See Debra Whiting Alexander, *Children Changed by Trauma* (Oakland, CA: New Harbinger Publication, 1999), 84.

95. Kimberly Smith [pseudo.], interview with the author, New Haven, CT, July 9, 2003.

96. Carolyn Yoder, *The Little Book of Trauma Healing* (Intercourse, PA: Good Books, 2005), 55–57.

97. For example, see Marie Fortune, "Forgiveness: The Last Step." Greg Jones offers an interesting Christian theological critique of forgiveness as a "last step." He argues, "For Christians, forgiveness is not a first or even a final 'step'; it is rather an embodied way of life." Christians learn this way of life, Jones continues, by taking part in the life of the church and the specific practices its members perform. Ultimately, forgiveness is an "invitation to imagine and embody a future, a future revealed in God's Kingdom that is not bound by the past or condemned to repeat it." See *Embodying Forgiveness: A Theological Analysis* (Grand Rapids, MI: Eerdmans, 1995), 89–90.

98. For example, see Debra Whiting Alexander, *Children Changed by Trauma*, 81–83.

99. Alexander, *Children Changed by Trauma*, 81–83.

4

Ecclesial Relations and the Healing of the Self

One trauma survivor who was abused as a child stated that her healing from this abuse began in the church she attended during her youth. When pressed to articulate how this church had provided a space in which she could begin to heal, the survivor at first found herself at a loss for words. After pondering the question for a minute, she decided that the church had enabled the beginning of her healing simply by being the church. She remarked, "To just be church—to just be community—it can make a huge difference."[1]

In the next three chapters I explore this somewhat ambiguous claim. It is important to understand, since the survivor does not stand alone in her experience. While many survivors either do not participate in religious communities or find them unhelpful, others report that religious groups play a role in their recovery.[2] But what exactly does it mean that the church can foster healing from trauma "simply by being the church"? On one level, it means that Christian communities can provide the most basic condition that trauma theorists identify as necessary for healing: supportive relationships. Although the church does not always succeed in creating such relationships, Christian theologians and lay persons have long considered this to be an essential part of its ministry.

Beyond this, however, lies a less obvious way in which Christian communities, simply by "being the church," sometimes contribute to the healing of traumatized persons. These communities have specific narratives—the narratives of the life, death, and resurrection of Jesus—that church members integrate into their identities over time as they perform concrete practices, such as breaking bread, sharing a common meal, and passing the peace. These narratives, when internalized through communal practices, can help form or reconstitute church members' identities in a way that transforms internalized, traumatic violence and integrates an element of nonviolence into their being.

To understand how this reconstitution of identities can happen in Christian communities, I explore correlations between the three phases of healing summarized in the previous chapter and Yoder's view of what it means for the church to be the church. In this chapter I consider how Yoder's description of ecclesial relations resonates with, and is challenged by, trauma scholars' accounts of supportive relationships. In chapter 5 I explore parallels between Yoder's use of narrative and trauma theorists' reflections on the role that narrative plays in the recovery process. In chapter 6 I then examine Yoder's view of the church as an eschatological community in light of trauma theorists' accounts of reconnecting with the present and imaging a better future. Taken as a whole, these chapters reconceptualize Christian nonviolence to include the transformation of internalized, traumatic violence through the communal enactment of a new identity.

In rethinking nonviolence in this way, it is crucial not to overestimate the assistance that Christian communities give to trauma survivors. Unfortunately, churches often fail survivors in many ways. For example, some women who endure domestic abuse are encouraged to submit to the violence by church teachings and structures that either explicitly or implicitly encourage acquiescence.[3] Religious leaders at times not only fail to assist trauma victims but also perpetrate trauma themselves, as in cases of clergy sexual abuse. In addition, many faith communities participate in broader societal denial about trauma by refusing to acknowledge its prevalence and impact.[4] Thus, in describing how the church may help trauma survivors to heal simply by being the church, I am not suggesting that this is something the church always does. Instead, I am proposing that this is something Christian communities are called to do. Put simply, they are called to provide a space in which traumatized persons can survive and flourish.

The creation of such a space is an integral part of the church's identity as a nonviolent community. If we take seriously Yoder's claim that nonviolence is the cornerstone of Christian faith and discipleship, as well as trauma theory's insight that violence can become embedded over time within people's bodies, minds, and souls, then it follows that transforming internalized, traumatic violence must constitute an essential part of Christian nonviolence (and an essential part of what it means for the church to be the church). While Christian communities may not consistently live into this part of their identity, they sometimes succeed in doing so. Analyzing how this success happens can heighten awareness within Christian communities of their potential to assist trauma survivors. This, in turn, may provide the knowledge and motivation that churches and their members need to offer such assistance on a more consistent basis.

While Yoder's writings provide useful resources for analyzing this dimension of Christian nonviolence, the next three chapters do not represent an uncritical embrace of his work. Yoder's theology provides a helpful starting place for the reconceptualization of nonviolence that I am developing, since he considers nonviolence integral to the church's identity and mission; as we have seen, however, he does not explicitly address internalized, traumatic violence. In each of the following chapters, my theological reflections thus begin with Yoder's writings but move beyond them. At times, I turn to the works of feminist and womanist theologians, who generally do not engage clinical accounts of trauma but nonetheless remain attentive to the ways in which overwhelming violence and structures of oppression affect individuals and communities over time. Their writings resonate in some ways with trauma studies and, therefore, provide useful resources for the reconceptualization of nonviolence that I am developing.

The analysis offered here does not constitute a systematic theology or a comprehensive account of the church's resources for healing. Instead, it presents some theological reflections which, though necessarily incomplete, generate insight into the possible resources that Christian communities can offer trauma survivors. Christian communities have long struggled with the reality of trauma, looking for ways to address the violence their members experience (and sometimes commit). However, they have not had the language and conceptuality of trauma studies to aid them in this task. Contemporary trauma studies, with its detailed description of trauma's effects, brings something new to theological reflection on nonviolence and healing. Its insights point toward an often-overlooked dimension of nonviolence and help to clarify how the church might enact it. This, in turn, makes it possible to understand better how Christian communities are not only sites of violence, but also sites of grace.

TRAUMA AND ECCLESIAL RELATIONS

The most basic way that Christian communities can help to foster recovery from trauma is by creating the relational conditions that make such recovery possible. Trauma theorists often observe that healing from traumatic violence does not take place in isolation; and Christian communities, like other communities, have potential to create the quality of relationships that enables healing from traumatization. To understand how this may happen, however, requires a more specific account of what such relationships look like in Christian communities and how they can be formed. This leads us to one central topic of ecclesiology: the nature of ecclesial relations and the social shape of the church. Yoder's work provides a helpful starting place for this analysis because it contends that part of what makes the church "church" is the way its members relate: how they speak with each other, how they listen to what others say, and how they interact on an ongoing basis. For Yoder, the church is not just a collection of individuals but a social organism or body in which each member needs and serves the other: "the whole is more than all of the parts, and . . . the interdependence of all is structured according to an already given plan, flexible and able to grow, but neither chaotic nor infinitely negotiable."[5]

In considering the nature of ecclesial relationships that Yoder describes, I focus on three related concepts he uses to talk about the character of Christian community. Yoder describes the church as a voluntary community that makes a confession of faith and commitment to discipleship the foundation of communal membership, an egalitarian community that values the gifts of each person, and a witnessing community that proclaims a message about God's kingdom to the broader society. While these three characteristics certainly do not describe the whole of his vision of ecclesial relations, I concentrate on them in particular because they open up topics that surface in trauma theorists' accounts of recovery—topics such as agency, power, and language. In examining each theme I first explore Yoder's interpretation, then consider how it might look from the perspective of trauma studies. This analysis of ecclesial relations from the perspective of trauma theory makes it possible to begin envisioning how the church may enact nonviolence by providing a space in which internalized, traumatic violence can be transformed through the reconstitution of church members' identities.

THE CHURCH AS VOLUNTARY COMMUNITY

In his ecclesiological writings, Yoder underscores the voluntary nature of the church.[6] When he uses this term, he clearly means more than the separation of church and state and freedom of expression in religious matters. As James McClendon observes, all churches in North America today are voluntary in the sense that there exists no state church and no law that makes one a member of any particular faith community.[7] For Yoder, the "voluntary" character of Christian community means, more specifically, that Christians choose to join the church because they have made a confession of faith in Jesus and a commitment to a life of discipleship. Given this emphasis on confession and commitment, he endorses the practice of adult baptism. Yoder insists that a person must enter the church not because they feel pressure to do so or because their parents have made this decision for them, but because they have heard and believed the gospel message and remain willing to accept the disciplines of the Christian life.[8]

On the surface, the language of voluntarism may seem to suggest that individuals make their decisions apart from the influences of others. As McClendon argues, however, the language of voluntarism need not imply this. Those who speak of voluntarism often acknowledge that our so-called free decisions are, in fact, informed (but not completely determined) by a variety of sources.[9] Thus, the decision to become part of the church is one that individuals make within a network of relationships and social contexts, including the Christian community. Since individuals can take part in the church before becoming members, the church may influence their decision to join in many ways. For example, it may offer preaching that evokes their belief, activities that inspire their interest and passion, and rituals that help them experience connection with the divine. In response to such practices, individuals may choose to make (or not make) a confession of faith and become members of the church.

Yoder suggests, however, that it is not only Christian communities that shape a person's decision to become part of the church but also God. While the language of voluntarism suggests that individual acts of faith are the foundation for the church, he contends that the church is also the result of God's work through the Spirit. This does not mean that the Christian community merely emerges from the sum of those decisions that are the Spirit's work. In Yoder's view, the church is not the product of a message in the way that "the crowd in the theater is the product of the reputation of the film."[10] Rather, God's work in history involves uniting people through the Spirit to form a new social humanity, and the church is called to exist as this new humanity into which people are inducted.[11] Individuals can choose to take up membership in the church, but their choices do not create it. Voluntarism thus means not only that those who choose to believe in Jesus and follow after him constitute the foundation of the church, but also that God's work through the church is the foundation of their choice.[12]

This complex relation between the individual, community, and divine that one finds in Yoder's work reveals that his theological framework does not offer an individualistic conception of "church." In his view, the church is a social body united by the confession of faith and commitment to discipleship that its members have made. Since all members have made this confession and commitment, they share a connection among themselves as well. Jesus serves as the common thread or "head" that holds the body together, such that one cannot have a relationship with him apart from one's relationships with the other members.[13] The union with Jesus that church members experience is, at the same time, a union with the other members of his body.

For Yoder, people establish this union with Jesus and his "body" partly through the community's enactment of relationships characterized by love. He states, "You can make people come to church, but you cannot make them love one another. The criterion of unfeigned love is, therefore, the index of the voluntary character of the fellowship."[14] This love entails a commitment to the well-being of others that is expressed, in part, through the offer of material support to those who need it.[15] In *Body Politics*, Yoder argues that the church's ministry involves the formation of economic community in which those who are materially privileged share their resources with those who are not. Theologically, he grounds this notion of economic sharing in the practice of breaking bread together.[16] In Yoder's view, Jesus and his disciples understood this practice to mean that they must share their day-to-day material sustenance. If one member of the church has concrete material needs, the others must strive to help fulfill them.

This offer of material support, however, does not alone constitute the essence of Christian love. Yoder indicates that love must entail spiritual nurturing as well, which communities can foster, in part, through reconciling dialogue. He describes this practice as "binding and loosing" and asserts that it has multiple applications. In one sense, binding and loosing is a process of reconciliation in which offenders are held accountable for their actions (binding) with the goal of being restored to the community (loosing).[17] In this practice, one member who has been offended by another confronts the offender in an effort to resolve the conflict constructively. In processing their conflicts, members learn communication skills, awareness, trust, and hope—in short, they build a community in which they can grow as persons. In addition, Yoder argues that it increases a person's self-esteem to know that others take their relationship seriously enough to seek reconciliation.[18] Yet, he cautions that not all communities can effectively practice this aspect of love. Reconciliation presumes a context of trust, which may not be present in communities in which members have not committed themselves to this standard.[19]

The voluntary nature of the church, then, presupposes not only that one makes a confession of faith in Jesus, but also that one embodies the love he enacted. For Yoder, this love that Christians are called to manifest is the Spirit's love expressed through their community: "The community's action is God's action."[20] Empowered by the Spirit, the church can live in faithful discipleship to Jesus as a community that, despite its brokenness, reveals God's grace. The voluntary character of the church thus underscores the notion that the church is a visible community, a new social reality that communicates a specific message about God's work in the world through its actions as well as its words.

From the perspective of trauma theory, Yoder's view of the church as a voluntary community that enacts relationships of love points to at least two ways in which the church may enable healing from trauma. First, his work calls Christian communities to create supportive contexts in which every member is cared for and affirmed. For survivors who have concrete needs, such a community can offer not only a physically secure space but also welcome relief from the material stresses that burden their daily lives. For example, consider a domestic violence survivor who has recently left her abuser but is struggling to make ends meet. The church that embodies the love Yoder describes would offer this survivor material assistance in whatever ways possible—perhaps by helping her to find a job, a place to live, and affordable child care. It would also provide a context in which she receives affirmation and care that she did not get in her home. By treating this survivor as a person who deserves respect and as an important member of the community, the church would create a space where she may come to believe that she is (and deserves to be) loved by others and by God.

Yoder's view of Christian love points to a second way in which the church may enable healing by underscoring two themes central to trauma scholars' accounts of recovery: agency and responsibility. Christian love, as he describes it, requires that each member of the community work to form and sustain relationships of accountability and trust.[21] In emphasizing the accountability and responsibility of each person, this vision of Christian community underscores the agentic potential of its members. This affirmation of their agency may help some survivors who were victimized by communities in which they did *not* choose to participate and in which their agency was undermined. For example, survivors born into abusive families may find it liberating to participate in a voluntary community that makes itself both responsible *for* its members and *to* them; within this context, unlike within their families, they have the power to call others to account. Moreover, some trauma survivors may find it empowering to take part in decision-making processes and to have the freedom to elect whether to dissent from or affirm the choices of the group. This emphasis on their responsibility to help build and sustain the church's structures and relationships underscores their agency by stressing that they can contribute to the larger good of the community.

At the same time, the rhetoric of voluntarism may prove problematic for other trauma survivors. Some survivors feel responsible for the sins they have suffered as well as for those they have committed. Used uncritically, the language of voluntarism might reinforce feelings of guilt and self-blame that may come with this strong sense of responsibility.[22] Underlying the notion of voluntary community is the assumption that people are empowered to make intentional decisions. While some theologians who talk about voluntarism do note that our choices are, to a certain extent, influenced by others, they maintain that these choices are not so influenced as to impair our ability to function as intentional agents.[23] Their language of voluntarism thus presumes an agency that is intact and whole rather than one that is compromised. As discussed in chapter 2, however, trauma theorists contend that while survivors often exercise agency in remarkable ways, they may also experience a loss of agency, a sense that they are unable to control their thoughts and emotions and to direct the course of their lives.

The concept of voluntary community can become more useful for trauma survivors if reconceptualized in a way that does not simply presume agency but instead explores how the church may help reconstitute agency when it has been diminished. From a theological perspective, this exploration can begin with a revised account of "binding and loosing."[24] Instead of focusing on the restoration of individuals who have offended others in the community, this account concentrates on how the church may help restore those who suffer from the effects of traumas they have experienced outside of the church. In this context, binding is recast as the process of tying together or integrating the fragmented self, and loosing as the self's release from the burdens imposed by traumatic harms. Binding thus includes the reconstitution of shattered agency, and loosing involves addressing both material obstacles to healing and trauma's psychological effects. I noted above that the church may help facilitate these dimensions of loosing by enacting the love Yoder describes. But what does binding look like from this viewpoint? How might Christian communities enable the integration of shattered agency?

On one level, it seems that binding can happen in much the same way as loosing: through the support of the Christian community. Recall that for many survivors, the healing of agency takes place over time in the context of healthy relationships. As they form attachments in which they receive respect and affirmation, survivors can gradually rebuild their sense of agency and capacity to make choices that promote their well-being. In light of this theoretical account of agency's reconstitution, one could argue that the church can facilitate the healing of agency, in part, by creating the kind of ecclesial relations that make this healing possible. For example, the church can enable "binding" by forming a hospitable community that openly welcomes all persons, treating them as individuals who matter. It can also facilitate the reconstitution of agency by building a participatory community that invites people to engage in church life—for instance, by serving as liturgical officers or taking part in decision-making processes. In addition, the church can contribute to the healing of shattered agency by being a socially active community that encourages its members to become involved in social justice efforts. Recall that some trauma survivors find that by working on behalf of others, they come to believe that they have the power to make a difference.

The healing of agency that may take place in Christian communities, however, does not happen solely through the efforts of the community or individual survivors. From a theological perspective, one can understand this experience of healing to derive, in part, from God's grace. This grace comes to the community through the work of the Spirit, who gathers the church and the people who constitute it. More precisely, one aspect of the work of grace is to form the church in which people with shattered agency are pulled together by the Spirit's love as manifest through the love of the community. Survivors and others in this community can experience this love in small ways—through the church's attempt to hear the voices of all its members, through its occasional preaching of a sermon that powerfully speaks to their fears and concerns, and through the warmth on the faces of strangers as they "pass the peace" on Sunday mornings.

Despite their many limitations and failures to attend to traumatized persons, then, Christian communities have the potential to enable spiritual growth and transformation. When they do, people can make the decision to become part of the church in a supportive context in which others remain committed to their well-being. Since individuals can certainly participate in the church before deciding to join, they may benefit from the resources of this community even if they are not members. For instance, the church that practices love as Yoder describes it would offer assistance and care to those who suffer violence even if they have not committed to join the church and to live the life of discipleship that this commitment entails. In addition, this community may show its respect for such survivors of violence by inviting them to actively participate in its life and worship. This invitation does not override their freedom or compel an affirmative response. The voluntary character of the church thus holds in tension the agency of the individual and the loving context of the community that is the condition of the possibility of the full exercise of that agency. By maintaining this tension, it points to one way in which traumatized persons may experience healing in a religious community.

THE CHURCH AS EGALITARIAN COMMUNITY

Based on his reading of the New Testament, Yoder articulates a vision of the church as an egalitarian community. He contends that Jesus formed a voluntary and egalitarian community in which a diverse group of people could live together in peace. In Yoder's view, this vision did not fade away after Jesus' death but rather continued in the life and writings of Paul. Yoder argues, for example, that Paul understood baptism as "the formation of a new people whose newness and togetherness explicitly relativize prior stratifications and classification. . . . [Its] first, ordinary meaning is egalitarian."[25] Similarly, he asserts that Paul's use of the body metaphor for Christian community is anti-hierarchical because it maintains that all members of this body are equally, though differently, empowered by the Spirit.[26]

When Yoder speaks of egalitarianism, he does not mean that everyone should be treated the same or that the church should have no leadership roles. Rather, he suggests that Christian communities must honor the value and contributions of each person. This means refusing to grant elevated status to those who come to the community with more power and instead attributing the most status to those who come with less.[27] When the church does this, it lives as the "new humanity on the way"—the part of the world that confesses and exemplifies the renewal to which the whole world is ultimately called.[28]

Yoder's work points to at least two important dimensions of egalitarianism. The first is power-sharing: Since not everyone comes to the church with the same access to social, political, and economic power, one task of egalitarian community is to implement structures and styles of leadership that share and multiply power rather than concentrate it in the hands of a few. Yoder indicates that Christian communities can accomplish this, in part, by performing specific practices derived from scripture that attend to the power dynamics within the church. He analyzes five practices that were central to the lives of early Christian communities—binding and loosing, baptism, eucharist, fullness of Christ, and rule of Paul—and that Yoder believes create and sustain egalitarian community by enabling power-sharing. For example, in the practice of universal ministry or fullness of Christ, the church honors the gifts of each member as enablements of the Spirit. By acknowledging that the Spirit equally empowers every person in the community, Christians can resist allowing a select few to accumulate power and embody instead Paul's vision of every-member empowerment.

Along similar lines, Yoder asserts that the church enacts power-sharing when it follows the "rule of Paul" in its worship or meetings. As he describes it, the rule of Paul is a procedure in which the Christian community discerns the Spirit's will by listening to what all who wish to speak—including those traditionally silenced—have to say.[29] This procedure has its theological roots in the conviction that there is God in every person. Since each person has a divinely imparted potential to hear the Spirit, each must have a chance to speak. More specifically, the rule of Paul relies on a model of consensus-building, which yields a decision only when the consensus becomes clear: "Until everyone with something to say has had the floor and until those who care have talked themselves out, the Spirit's will is not clearly known."[30]

In addition to power-sharing, Yoder's work indicates that reciprocity represents a second integral dimension of egalitarian relationships. He describes binding and loosing, for example, as a social practice that requires dialogue and deliberation undertaken in a spirit of mutual trust.[31] Forgiveness—another integral part of this practice—both presumes and creates goodwill between all parties in the relationship. For Yoder, then, one marker of egalitarianism is that the lines of care and consideration are not unilinear. As a voluntary community, the church must establish and sustain relationships in which each member both gives and receives—relationships in which every person embodies the reliability and faithfulness that makes mutual trust possible and in which every person makes their own contributions and benefits from the contributions of others.

Yoder's vision of the church as an egalitarian community that shares power may prove useful for some survivors who struggle with disempowerment. Recall that Yoder believes that power is part of God's good creation and therefore is good, though it can be used in destructive ways.[32] Since power is essentially good, Christians are called not to divest themselves of power but to equally empower all persons in their communities. If the church enacts power-sharing as Yoder envisions it, then it may provide a context in which survivors begin to reclaim their power. Trauma theorists argue that an important source of empowerment is trust, care, love, and freedom; and Yoder's view of the church as voluntary and egalitarian portrays it as a community that can offer these gifts.

Furthermore, Yoder's sense that the church should enact reciprocal relationships of trust and care may also resonate with trauma survivors who experience disempowerment. One abuse survivor, for example, offers a personal account of the ways she has benefited from participating in a church that sought to embody egalitarian relationships marked by reciprocity. This community arranged its chairs in a circle and exchanged reciprocal blessings, simple practices which led her to have a more positive experience of the church than she had in previous periods of her life. Having attended churches of different denominations throughout her life, she had always remained troubled by the ways in which these communities invested power and authority in particular individuals or in the church as a whole. For her, the hierarchical structures of the church had reinforced feelings of disempowerment. Attending a church that consciously sought to enact reciprocal trust and care enabled her to begin the long process of reclaiming her sense of power and agency, a crucial part of her healing.[33]

In *Trauma and Recovery*, Herman identifies specific ways that reciprocal relationships facilitate healing for some survivors. Rather than analyzing the structure and practice of religious communities, she considers the dynamics of another form of community: survivor groups. In her view, any kind of relationship can provide "mutually enhancing interaction," but this occurs most powerfully within a group. She writes,

> Groups provide the possibility not only of mutually rewarding relationships but also of collective empowerment. Group members approach one another as peers and equals. Though each is suffering and in need of help, each also has something to contribute. The group requisitions and nurtures the strengths of its members. As a result, the group as a whole has the capacity to bear and integrate traumatic experience that is greater than that of any individual member, and each member can draw upon the shared resources of the group to foster her own integration.[34]

Some survivors find that the mutual exchange of stories that takes place in these groups enables them to identify strengths in themselves that they see in others. Others discover that the reciprocal exchange of love, trust, care and freedom helps them rebuild their capacity for self-care and ability to cultivate healthy relationships. As one individual says, "I'm better able to take in the love of others, and this is cyclical in allowing me to be more loving to myself, and then to others."[35]

While Yoder's understanding of the church seems compatible in some ways with the communal dynamics Herman describes, one aspect of his vision may elicit a negative response from those concerned about trauma. In *The Politics of Jesus*, he speaks of reciprocal relationships, as does Herman; but he does so in the context of a discussion of "revolutionary subordination," a concept he derives from New Testament passages in which Paul calls on slaves, women, and children to subordinate themselves to their masters, husbands, and parents (and vice versa). Yoder finds Paul's call to subordination revolutionary because it has reciprocal form: It not only calls on those with lesser status to voluntarily accept their positions, but also demands that those with more status bow to their subjects.[36] In his view, this call to mutual subordination transforms existing power relations by requiring those "at the top" to refrain from exercising power over others, and by affirming that those "at the bottom" are moral agents capable of transforming domination into willing servanthood and thereby living without hate and resentment.

While this concept of mutual subordination may illuminate one way that communities can resist the current social order without actively perpetrating violence, it proves less helpful for discerning how they may contribute to the healing of selves who are sites of violence. The claim that empowerment comes through subordination makes little sense in many situations of trauma, especially those that involve interpersonal harm. When survivors subordinate themselves to abusive others, they often experience further disempowerment. To be fair, Yoder does not describe subordination to the powers as passive acquiescence or obedience to unjust circumstances. Instead, he distinguishes subordination from subjection, which he claims "carries a connotation of being thrown down and run over," and submission, which he says has a "connotation of passivity."[37] However, the rhetoric of subordination can be easily misunderstood to mean subjection or submission, and it therefore risks recapitulating patterns that perpetuate violence and oppression. For this reason, the language of willing subordination is not the best choice for describing the relationships that the church ideally would embody.

Instead, the language of egalitarianism, power-sharing, and reciprocity is better suited for this task. While the church does not have all the resources that survivors need, it can help foster recovery by forming egalitarian relationships in which individuals offer to each other gifts necessary for healing: love, care, trust, and freedom. When Christian communities honor the worth of each person and value their contributions, they create and sustain relationships that challenge the hierarchical character of the powers. In so doing, they offer a space in which those who experience disempowerment can begin to reclaim their power. Christian communities may participate in this way, even if only to a small degree, in the transformation of traumatic violence through healing.

THE CHURCH AS WITNESSING COMMUNITY

In "A People in the World," Yoder observes that the sixteenth-century Anabaptist Menno Simons identified the concept of witness as one of the central marks of the church. In a polemical discussion, he compares Menno's view of the church's witness—its proclamation of a message to the broader society—to the different perspectives of Ulrich Zwingli and Caspar Schwenckfeld. Yoder argues that Zwingli understands the Christian witness as a means of achieving social change; for him, witnessing entails addressing relevant issues from a Christian perspective in order to favorably alter the structures of society. By contrast, Schwenckfeld believes that Christian witness should focus not on transforming the social order but on convincing individuals to accept the gospel message. Yoder contends that these two perspectives have something in common: Both dilute the church's witness, either by defining it in the terms of the wider society or by focusing solely on how it affects individuals. Rejecting these positions, he argues in favor of Menno's view, which he believes takes seriously the need for social change and individual piety but does not make either of these concerns the unique focus. Yoder contends that for Menno, Christian witness focuses on presenting a message without compromise in the face of a hostile world. The crucial factor is not whether the witness facilitates social change or individual conversions but whether the church continues to faithfully proclaim its message, even when it encounters strong resistance.[38]

For Yoder, the message that the church is called to present has its roots in Jesus' proclamation of God's kingdom. In his life, Jesus pronounced that this kingdom had drawn near; in his death and resurrection, the kingdom was inaugurated. Yoder argues that the church, in its witnessing function, must communicate this message about God's kingdom to the broader culture not only through what it says but even more through what it does. Specifically, the church proclaims its message by living as a community that manifests in its own life the way Jesus lived and died.[39] This means that the church must have the form of a visible and distinct social reality, a voluntary and egalitarian community that embodies Jesus' nonviolent resistance to the powers. In witnessing to God's love as revealed in Jesus, the church does not act as an instrument of the kingdom, bringing it into this world.[40] Instead, it represents in its social life the shape of God's kingdom. The church proclaims and reveals to the world the inauguration of a new age—one that profoundly shapes reality on a social and economic level.[41]

Yoder contends that participating in this new order means living an eschatological existence. The Christian community is called to witness to the message about God's kingdom even in the face of the powers' continued destruction; in so doing, this community takes it on faith that God will make things come out right. Given that the church puts its hope and trust into God's acting, the key criterion of its witness is not immediate effectiveness but conformity to the new order inaugurated by Jesus. This criterion of conformity requires Christians to focus not on reordering society or revitalizing the soul but on restructuring the life of the Christian community. Only then does the church faithfully embody its eschatological witness in the world.[42]

Yoder argues, however, that this integrity comes with a price. In witnessing to the world, the Christian community exists in the middle of the old order and in contradiction to it. Therefore, its social nonconformity at times will be costly: "To follow after Christ is not simply to learn from him, but also to share his destiny."[43] Yoder says that suffering is not itself redemptive and martyrdom is not a goal the church should seek; however, he also believes that the church must accept that its witness at times will generate painful confrontation with the powers. As he puts it, "The cross is not a recipe for resurrection. Suffering is not a tool to make people come around, nor a good in itself. But the kind of faithfulness that is willing to accept evident defeat rather than complicity with evil is . . . aligned with the ultimate triumph of the Lamb."[44]

In emphasizing that the church, in its witnessing function, must concentrate first and foremost on its faithfulness to Jesus, Yoder does not suggest that the present is just a time of looking to the future for the fulfillment of God's plan. Rather, he argues that the eschaton, though not yet fully consummated, has entered history in the incarnation and work of Jesus, and the Christian community participates in it when it embodies the character of God's love as revealed in Jesus. To indicate this present quality of the eschaton, Yoder speaks of two overlapping aeons that exist simultaneously. The "old" aeon, characterized by sin and rebellion against God, points backward to life apart from Jesus; the "new" aeon, characterized by the reign of Christ, points forward "to the fullness of the kingdom of God, of which it is a foretaste."[45] According to Yoder, each aeon has a "social manifestation": the old in the "world," and the new in the body of Christ.[46]

In Yoder's view, the new aeon involves a "radical break with the old" but does not replace or destroy the old.[47] Instead, the new social reality that Jesus established offers an alternative to the old order. Yoder argues that according to the New Testament,

> the essential change which has taken place is not within the realm of the old aeon, vengeance and the state, where there is really no change; it is rather that the new aeon revealed in Christ takes primacy over the old, explains the meaning of the old, and will finally vanquish the old. The state did not change with the coming of Christ; what changed was the coming of the new aeon which proclaimed the doom of the old one.[48]

Through its creation of a new social reality and the rejection of violence, the church participates in the new aeon. In so doing, it lives as an eschatological community that bears witness to Jesus, manifesting the life God intends for all.

How might we analyze this understanding of the church's witness from the viewpoint of trauma studies? On the one hand, Yoder's description of the content of the church's witness may provide some trauma survivors with a word of hope. The message about God's kingdom that is central to this witness offers a vision of an abundant and life-giving future that may temper the fear and disillusionment that results from their traumas. This vision of a different future, a future not dominated by traumatic violence, may represent a particularly helpful resource for survivors who suffer from a foreshortened sense of the future that renders them unable to think much about what is to come, let alone envision it in positive ways (I address this matter further in chapter 6).

On the other hand, Yoder does not explicitly extend the concept of witnessing to address an important dimension that trauma theory identifies. He focuses on how the church can witness to the world about Jesus' proclamation of the kingdom, but he does not talk about how the church can witness to the suffering its own members experience. He does implicitly point to this dimension of witnessing when he claims that Christian communities must bear witness to Jesus and to the kingdom by continuing Jesus' ministry in the world—a ministry that entailed caring for those in need and creating life-giving relationships. But trauma theory encourages us to address this dimension of witnessing explicitly and with reference to trauma's specific effects. It requires us to ask: How might Christian communities bear witness to the traumatized in their midst?

Scripture contains multiple stories that illustrate one way these communities may bear such witness: by providing a context in which people can express their grievances to God and ask for God's help. For example, Job becomes angry with God and demands the right to argue his case before God when he loses his wealth, posterity, and health. Similarly, Moses cries out to God when the Israelites are stuck in the wilderness without water.[49] And the psalter of Lamentations expresses the agony of the people of Jerusalem and offers a cry to God for mercy after the Babylonians destroy Jerusalem.[50]

Drawing on these passages, one could offer a broader concept of witnessing that includes not only the proclamation of an undiluted message to the surrounding society, but also the voicing of one's own pain (and the pain of others) to God.

This broader understanding of witness is vital to any view of Christian community that seeks to respond to the suffering that results from traumatic violence. Recall that some trauma survivors experience grief and anger at God, and expressing this anger in constructive ways constitutes an important part of their healing process. One way to express grief and anger constructively is to protest the injustice of one's situation to God. For some trauma survivors, having permission to register their complaints with God gives them a way to mourn their losses. It may also enable them to rethink their images of the divine. Rather than viewing God as one who demands unwavering devotion, they may see God as one who can withstand questioning and who listens to their complaints. The book of Exodus, for example, describes God as one who hears the cries of the Israelites enslaved in Egypt and responds by bringing them to Canaan (Exodus 3: 7–8). The Psalms portray God as hearing people's cries and responding with concern (Psalms 6: 8).

An understanding of witnessing that more fully attends to the suffering that results from trauma must include not only the proclamation of one's grievances to God and God's reception of them, but also the church's response to the stories of pain that traumatized persons tell. One place to begin reconceptualizing witnessing in this way is with Yoder's claim that the church carries out its witness by attending to the structures of its own social life. For the church to form a community that bears witness to trauma survivors, it must intentionally work to create the kind of relational conditions in which the stories of its members—stories of violence and loss as well as of joy—can be told and heard. The voluntary and egalitarian character of the church is essential to this task. As a voluntary community, the church welcomes but does not compel its members to share their stories; as an egalitarian community, the church seeks to form relations in which the voices of all people are valued and affirmed. The voluntary and egalitarian church can thus witness to Jesus' proclamation of the kingdom by listening and responding to the suffering that people experience in the present, not only the suffering that comes from a chosen life of social nonconformity, but also the suffering that results from unwanted experiences of violence and oppression.

Too often in the experience of trauma survivors, however, the church does not bear witness in this way. To maintain their sense of safety and predictability, both clergy and lay persons often deny the prevalence of trauma or respond to stories of violence with indifference or judgment.[51] At other times, they communicate in subtle ways that they do not want to hear about the traumas people have experienced. For example, a church may not include a time in its worship to voice concerns and ask for prayer requests. It may demonstrate an unwillingness to hear about trauma through preaching that refuses to allow the reality of violence to challenge theological accounts of God's justice, grace, sin, and redemption. In some instances, churches also communicate a lack of willingness to hear about trauma by not offering respectful silence when trauma does receive mention, responding instead with words designed to direct the conversation toward "happier" matters. To witness more effectively to the suffering of trauma survivors, then, the church must continually critique its own social life to discern the ways in which it fails to welcome narratives of trauma.

The church may fail to witness to the reality of trauma because, as Dori Laub suggests, the cost of witnessing can be high. Bearing witness to traumatic violence involves exposing oneself to terror and tremendous loss, and while this exposure remains crucial to the survivor's healing, it places the hearer at risk.[52] As we saw in chapter 2, those who hear about trauma are not affected in the same way as those who experience trauma firsthand; however, they are affected, often in profoundly unsettling ways. Hearing about trauma can destabilize one's worldview, calling into question basic assumptions about God, evil, and the meaning of life. It can also alter the ways in which both survivors and their witnesses view certain aspects of religious life. For instance, Christians who witness to others' traumas may come to see the community's practices and liturgies in a different light. They may come to view the eucharist as a recollection of trauma rather than a celebration of God's grace. Or, they may find that hymns which speak of Jesus' blood evoke memories about violence and loss rather than promise and new life. In the context of trauma, old traditions and words can take on new meaning.

The presence of witnesses who open themselves to this destabilizing impact of stories about trauma, however, is necessary for survivors to heal. As Herman observes, healing requires the creation of a community of survivors and their witnesses: "It cannot be reiterated too often: *no one can face trauma alone*."[53] When the church lives as a voluntary and egalitarian community that bears witness to the reality of the suffering that traumatized individuals experience, it creates a space in which survivors do not have to deal with their traumas entirely on their own. These traumas become part of the church's life, and the whole community must then face them together.

As we have seen, however, facing trauma together is a difficult task. The analysis of ecclesial relations that I have offered in this chapter only begins to suggest ways in which Christian communities can assist traumatized persons in their recovery process. By creating a set of relationships that help to reconstitute shattered agency, by empowering those who have limited power, and by witnessing to profound human suffering, Christian communities may help trauma survivors to transform some of the effects of traumatization with which they struggle. I have been arguing that this transformation of trauma's effects (internal violence) represents an integral dimension of Christian nonviolence. But for traumatized persons to move further in their recovery process, and for the church to enact nonviolence more fully, much more needs to happen. In the next chapter, I explore a piece of this "more" by theologically reflecting on the second phase of healing that many trauma theorists describe: creating a narrative of the trauma.

NOTES

1. Jane Miller [pseudo.], conversation with the author, New Haven, CT, July 7, 2003.

2. Alexander McFarlane and Bessel van der Kolk, "Trauma and Its Challenge to Society," 25.

3. Christine E. Gudorf, *Victimization: Examining Christian Complacency* (Philadelphia: Trinity Press International, 1992), 90–93.

4. See Marie Fortune, *Sexual Violence: The Unmentionable Sin* (Cleveland: Pilgrim Press, 1983).

5. Yoder, *Body Politics*, ix.

6. For example, see Yoder, "A People in the World" and "The Hermeneutics of Peoplehood" in *The Royal Priesthood*.

7. McClendon, "The Voluntary Church in the Twenty-First Century," in *The Believers Church: A Voluntary Church*, ed. by William H. Brackney (Ontario, ON: Pandora Press, 1998), 180.

8. Those who are members of churches that practice infant baptism may still understand their tradition as "voluntary." From this perspective, the practice of infant baptism allows others to make the decision for the child to become an official church member; however, this child still chooses at a later time whether to live into this decision and become an active participant in the church.

9. McClendon, "Voluntary Church in the Twenty-First Century," 180.

10. Yoder, "A People in the World," 74.

11. See Yoder, "A People in the World," 73–75.

12. See George Vandervelde, "Believers Church Ecclesiology as Ecumenical Challenge," in *The Believers Church: A Voluntary Church*, 206.

13. Yoder speaks of Christ as the head in *Body Politics*, 53.

14. Yoder, "A People in the World," 82.

15. Yoder does not explicitly connect his statements on love with the sharing of material sustenance, but his work leaves room for such an interpretation. See *Body Politics*, chapters 1 and 2.

16. See Yoder, *Body Politics*, 14–27.

17. Yoder, "Binding and Loosing," *The Royal Priesthood*, 323–58 and *Body Politics*, 1–13.

18. Yoder, *Body Politics*, 8.

19. Yoder, *Body Politics*, 5.

20. Yoder, *Body Politics*, 3.

21. Yoder, *Body Politics*, 5.

22. For an account of the role that the themes of responsibility and agency played in one trauma survivor's healing process, see Rebecca, Lea Nicoll Kramer, and Susan A. Lakey, "Spirit Song: The Use of Christian Healing Rites in Trauma Recovery," *Treating Abuse Today* 5 and 6 (November/December 1995 and January/February 1996): 39–47.

23. For example, see the essays by McCLendon and Vandervelde in *The Believers Church*.

24. This constructive reworking of binding and loosing does not focus on forgiveness, partly because forgiveness represents too complex a matter to adequately address in such a brief space.

25. Yoder, *Body Politics*, 33.

26. Yoder, *Body Politics*, 55.

27. Yoder, *Body Politics*, 50.

28. Yoder, *Body Politics*, 78; Yoder, "The New Humanity as Pulpit and Paradigm," in *For the Nations*, 50.

29. Yoder, *Body Politics*, 69.

30. Yoder, *Body Politics*, 68.

31. Yoder, *Body Politics*, 6.

32. Yoder, *The Politics of Jesus*, 154.

33. Sally Morgan [pseudo.], personal conversation, New Haven, CT, July 8, 2003.

34. Herman, *Trauma and Recovery*, 216.

35. Qtd. in Herman, *Trauma and Recovery*, 216.

36. Yoder, *The Politics of Jesus*, 177.

37. Yoder, *The Politics of Jesus*, 172.

38. Yoder, "A People in the World," 84.

39. Yoder, "A People in the World," 74.

40. Yoder, "Discerning the Kingdom of God in the World," in *For the Nations*, 240.

41. See Reinhard Hütter, "The Church: Midwife of History or Witness of the Eschaton?" 45.

42. See Yoder, "A People in the World," 86–91.

43. Yoder, *The Politics of Jesus*, 124.

44. Yoder, *The Politics of Jesus*, 238.

45. Yoder, "If Christ Is Truly Lord," in *The Original Revolution*, 58–59; *The Politics of Jesus*, 186.

46. Yoder, "If Christ Is Truly Lord," 58.

47. Yoder, "If Christ Is Truly Lord," 58.

48. Yoder, "If Christ Is Truly Lord," 62.

49. Exodus 15:25.

50. Lamentations 2:1–22.

51. See Marie Fortune, *The Unmentionable Sin*, and Carolyn Holderread Heggen, *Sexual Abuse in Christian Homes and Churches* (Scottdale, PA: Herald Press, 1993).

52. Laub, "Bearing Witness," *Testimony*, 72.

53. Herman, *Trauma and Recovery*, 153.

5

Performing the Narratives of Jesus

One trauma survivor described her life as an "ongoing story—but not in the usual sense."[1] She explained that the story of her life, unlike the stories she read to her children, contained gaps and holes—places where chapters seemed missing and pieces did not fit together. In describing her life story as broken and disjunctive, this survivor echoed the claim of some trauma theorists that trauma can make it difficult for individuals to form an ongoing, personal narrative that gives them a sense of continuity and coherence. In chapters 2 and 3 I explored how trauma can resist being integrated into one's narrative, as well as the role that narrative plays in healing when survivors incorporate their traumas into their life stories by describing them in words. Moving beyond this theoretical account, I now develop theological reflections on this second phase of healing from trauma. These reflections add another dimension to the exploration of how the church may help foster healing simply by "being the church."

Yoder's view of Christian community and discipleship indicates that part of what it means for the church to "be the church" is to embody and internalize particular narratives—the narratives of Jesus' life, death, and resurrection. Yoder suggests that in the church, Christians integrate these narratives into their identities over time. Through their practices, they place themselves within the ongoing story of Jesus' life, such that his story becomes theirs as well. When viewed from the perspective of trauma studies, this relationship between narrative and identity formation in his work raises the questions: In what ways might the specific narratives that the church enacts contribute to the recovery of traumatized persons? What resources can the church's performance of these narratives offer to survivors who struggle with trauma's ongoing effects?

A fruitful place to begin addressing these questions is with the multifaceted nature of the narrative. The story of Jesus that Christianity proclaims and embodies has as one of its central moments an event of trauma, his crucifixion; however, this trauma does not completely dominate the broader narrative. Christian theology at its best gives equal weight and salvific significance to all aspects of Jesus' existence. The story of his death is held within the narratives of his life and resurrection, and within the much broader narrative of the world that spans from the beginning to the end of time. For some traumatized persons, this multifaceted narrative may foster healing by providing a framework that recontextualizes (but does not deny or minimize) their trauma. The trauma then no longer functions as the one experience that defines their life but as part of a bigger story or ongoing narrative. Thus, as Christians insert their own lives into this narrative, they put their traumas into a broader framework that both recognizes the reality of this violence and offers some hope for a different future, one not dominated by trauma.

This narrative into which Christians insert their lives, of course, presents potential difficulties for trauma survivors as well as possible resources for healing. On the one hand, part of what may prove so powerful for some survivors about the narrative that the church proclaims is precisely that it contains a story of trauma. When Christians enact the narrative they remember this story, which may enable them to recall their own traumas and place them within a broader framework, one that holds together their shattered fragments of memory. On the other hand, some theologians worry that the narratives of Jesus—in particular, their story of the cross—may seem to valorize suffering or evoke painful memories that re-traumatize survivors.[2] These concerns are not unwarranted, especially since many traumatized persons do not experience healing through their participation in Christian communities. As discussed in chapter 2, some find that their traumas raise such disturbing theological questions that they simply cannot turn to the church as a possible source of support; their experience of God's apparent absence or silence in the face of their suffering alienates them from religious traditions and communities.[3] In describing the church's resources for recovery, then, I do not deny the potential difficulties with its narratives but simply explore ways in which the church's performance of them may assist survivors who find that they do benefit from their life and worship in Christian community. Such exploration might encourage these communities to think more deeply about how traumatized persons respond to their practices, and how they can create contexts in which healing will more likely occur.

As I have argued throughout this book, attentiveness to the dynamics of traumatization within the church and its members constitutes an integral part of Christian nonviolence. Christian nonviolence includes the transformation of internalized, traumatic violence, and the church's communal enactment of the narratives of Jesus can play an integral role in this transformation. On their own, however, the biblical narratives of Jesus do not facilitate healing from trauma; these narratives become a possible resource for recovery only when traumatized persons take part in a community that internalizes them through its life and worship. Yoder's view of the narratives of Jesus and their relation to Christian practices gives us insight into how this internalization may take place. I begin, then, by turning to this aspect of his work.

NARRATIVE AND PRACTICES IN YODER'S THEOLOGY

The description of Yoder's ecclesiology and social ethics offered in chapter 1 indicates that narrative plays a key role in his theological vision. Recall that for Yoder, it is not the general category of narrative that is most important but the particular narratives of the life, death, and resurrection of Jesus.[4] In his view, the church's identity and mission are defined by these narratives; the gospels provide the norm for what the church should be and do. More specifically, scripture establishes a norm of nonviolence for the church by revealing that Jesus embodied a social-political-ethical stance of nonviolent resistance in relation to the powers and principalities. When the church embodies this stance in its own life, it "re-narrates" Jesus' story by manifesting his way of peace and justice.[5] Yoder indicates that the church manifests the way of Jesus not only by verbally proclaiming his story but also by enacting it. Christian discipleship, then, has a performative dimension: Christians follow Jesus and come to truly know him only when they place themselves within the gospel narratives and act out their commands.[6]

Yoder's understanding of Christian practices clarifies how the church enacts scripture. In his view, practices are what Christians do when they gather for reasons derived from their faith. They are social processes, activities in which the church comes together to carry out common tasks, such as making decisions and dealing with matters of power and rank.[7] As such, practices provide one way church members interact with each other and build ecclesial relations. Through their enactment of concrete practices, Christians form a particular kind of community and cultivate the skills necessary to live as faithful disciples. They do not, however, do this entirely on their own. Yoder asserts that practices involve both divine and human action. More precisely, they are "actions of God, in and with, through and under what men and women do."[8]

Yoder's work suggests that by performing the practices Jesus embodied, Christians place themselves within the biblical narratives and act out his story. When they gather to share a common meal, hold meetings in which all may speak, and reconcile their conflicts with one another, they act out the ongoing story of Jesus' life. In doing so, they integrate themselves into this story, such that they become "characters" who are "crafted" by the biblical texts.[9] As Christians shape their lives around this story that they hear and tell, it becomes theirs as well, an integral part of who they are. More specifically, the story of Jesus comes to inform the ways Christians perceive and respond to reality: It comes to shape how they think, act, speak, and make decisions.

By pointing to this performative dimension of discipleship, Yoder opens up the possibility that in Christian community people's identities can be formed by the biblical narratives. His work, however, does not suggest merely that the identities of individual Christians are formed in the church. If the church is, as Yoder suggests, a mutually interdependent social organism or social body, then its communal re-narration of Jesus' story shapes not only the identities of the individuals who help to constitute the church but also the identity of the Christian community as a whole. When the church gathers to perform practices derived from the narratives of Jesus, it participates in Jesus' life and has its identity reconstituted in him, making the body of Christ visible in the world. Yoder states, "Where [practices] are happening, the people of God is real in the world."[10]

Yoder's view of the relation between narrative and identity formation both resonates with and diverges from the insights of contemporary trauma studies. Like many trauma scholars, Yoder understands narrative to be central to the construction of identity; in his view, it shapes and defines our sense of ourselves, others, and the world around us. But whereas trauma scholars concentrate on the role that one's individual life story plays in forming one's identity, Yoder's work points to ways in which communal narratives can help to construct our identities as well. This has important implications for how we think about healing from trauma. As we have seen, trauma scholars claim that healing requires placing the traumatic experience into a narrative framework that contains the story of one's individual life. Yoder's work suggests the possibility that there exist larger, shared narratives—for example, the narratives of Jesus—into which survivors' stories can be incorporated and in which they can be transformed.

Trauma theorists' reflections on healing clarify how this integration of one's own narrative into the biblical story might help to foster recovery for some trauma survivors. Recall their claim that narrating the trauma and placing it within a broader framework is essential to healing because traumatic experiences often lack temporal and spatial location.[11] Overwhelming and incomprehensible, they have a timeless quality that severs their connection to "ordinary" experiences. In their timelessness, traumatic events resist integration and thus lack closure, continuing to recirculate into the present through flashbacks and other intrusive symptoms.[12] Narrating the trauma (and thereby placing it within a broader framework of memory and meaning) can stop this recirculation by giving the experience closure, a definite location in space and time.[13]

Not all narratives, however, provide resources that foster the healing and integration of the self. For example, narratives that contain only stories of horror and abuse do not facilitate healing. The placement of one's trauma into a larger narrative can transform the effects of trauma only if this narrative contextualizes the trauma within a framework that both acknowledges the reality of the violence and offers some hope for a better future. More specifically, the narrative must contain resources that temper the survivors' fear and disillusionment with a sense of hope and renewal, such that the trauma and its effects no longer define the whole of their existence.

To better understand how the survivors' placement of their own stories within the particular narratives of Jesus might help to foster their recovery from trauma—and how it also sometimes might fall short of this goal—requires looking at the content of these narratives. What, specifically, do the narratives say that might assist some trauma survivors? Which aspects of the story into which Christians integrate themselves through their practices might facilitate a recontextualization of their traumas that fosters healing and hope? And which aspects might be problematic for some survivors?

RE-EXAMINING THE NARRATIVES OF JESUS

When assessing the narratives of Jesus in relation to trauma, it is difficult to simply characterize some of its aspects as "helpful" and others as "harmful." The same dimensions of the church's narratives that assist one survivor may function as a stumbling block for another, partly due to the differing social contexts in which these narratives are encountered, the lack of uniformity among survivors' responses to their traumas, and the multiple ways in which individuals and communities can enact and interpret the narratives. While identifying potential resources for healing within the gospel narratives thus is a complex task, we can make some general remarks about this matter, beginning with scripture's descriptions of Jesus' life. As Yoder observes, a central focus of the gospels is Jesus' embodiment of a new vision of positive, abundant relationships in which all persons enjoy the benefits of just and peaceful community. These texts indicate that his ministry of creating this community involved reaching out to the marginalized, healing those with physical and psychological illness, and demanding the transformation of the status quo to make life more equally abundant.

When the church conforms (albeit imperfectly) to the vision of human life that Jesus proclaimed, it integrates itself into his story and is thereby shaped by the narratives of his ministry of righting relations and opposing injustice. As Christians re-narrate or enact the story of Jesus' life through their practices, they become people formed not only by their individual past and present but also by a vision that is inherently communal—one that includes Jesus' resistance to the powers, his call to right relatedness, and his love and compassion. In integrating themselves into a narrative that offers such a vision of wholeness and transformation, Christians locate their individual stories within a broader narrative framework. As they do so, their identities come to be defined not only by the stories of their individual lives, but also by the communal narratives that the church's members share—narratives that contain not only images of brokenness but also a positive vision of healing and hope. For some trauma survivors, this integration of their own stories into this larger, shared framework may help counter the isolation and totalizing despair that their traumatic experiences engendered.

The view of healing that I am developing, however, may appear problematic for some traumatized persons. I am suggesting that the reconstruction of identities which takes place through the church's practices can help to heal the traumatized self; however, the communal narratives that the church performs in these practices has the story of the cross as one of its central moments.[14] Thus, the Christian community enacts the identity of one whose life culminates in an event of traumatic violence. In its life and worship, the church invokes this trauma in many ways. For example, when Christians perform the Eucharist, they remember Christ's wounded body by describing the night of his death and repeating the biblical refrain: "This is my body, broken for you." Similarly, when they baptize new members, Christians say that the one being baptized "dies and rises" with Christ. What might it mean for traumatized persons to enact this story of one who was tortured on a cross before being raised from the dead? Would this performance be one that heals, or would it induce yet another mimetic replay of their traumas?

Many feminist and womanist theologians point out ways in which the symbol of the cross has functioned to generate mimetic reproductions of violence.[15] The cross, in their analysis, has often been used to create a social environment in which some people have been forced to bear the violence of their culture; their enduring this violence has then been seen as redemptive for the culture as a whole. In light of this, some feminist and womanist theologians suggest that the symbol of the cross cannot heal or redeem. Delores Williams, for example, argues that redemption has to do not with the cross but with God, through Jesus' life, "giving humankind the ethical thought and practice upon which to build positive, productive quality of life."[16] Drawing on her work, one might conclude that ritually performing a narrative that has the cross at its center inevitably contributes to the creation of conditions that produce subjects who suffer violence and mimetically reproduces violence in those who have endured it.

While recognizing the helpfulness of such critiques that point out ways in which the symbol of the cross can be (and often has been) used to harm and oppress individuals and communities, I suggest that the communal embodiment of a story that has the cross at its center, in some circumstances, can be healing and redemptive. In her study of the meaning of the cross in African American religious experience, Joanne Terrell argues that some communities which endure violence and oppression do turn to the cross as a source of hope and empowerment. In particular, many early Christian martyrs and enslaved Africans embraced the symbol of the cross because they saw in this symbol a reflection of their own suffering and an affirmation of their innocence.[17] While the situations of the martyrs and enslaved Africans were fundamentally different—the former were persecuted for their faith, which they had the option to deny; the latter were persecuted for the color of their skin, which they could not renounce—both groups found in the cross a source of solace and strength. Thus, Terrell refuses to deny the redemptive power of cross. She argues instead that the cross is "about God's love for humankind in a profound sense" and that "there *is* power in the blood, even in the *name* of Jesus."[18]

Yet discerning how to speak of this empowering potential in a way that does not replicate oppressive patterns of thinking and acting is a difficult task. One can guard against this replication by affirming two points. First, God does not sanction violence (against Jesus or us) or want people to experience violence and oppression. Second, our victimization and the suffering it engenders are not redemptive. In Yoder's words, the "cross is not a recipe for resurrection. Suffering is not a tool to make people come around, nor a good in itself."[19] As Terrell suggests, however, denying the redemptive power of our victimization does not require us to deny the redemptive power of the death of one who was both human and divine.[20] Those who suffer from experiences of victimization can be redeemed by his death, although not in isolation from the other aspects of his existence.[21] The life, death, and resurrection of Jesus together can redeem human beings, including those who suffer from trauma (and those who perpetrate it).

But to articulate how this redemption can take place and its relation to trauma healing requires offering an interpretation of the cross that is rhetorically sensitive to the experiences and needs of traumatized persons. As Williams rightly observes, traditional theories of atonement have often been used to perpetuate rather than transform oppression and violence. Given the diversity of ways in which theologians have understood the cross, we must ask: How might the claims Christians make about the cross affect trauma survivors in particular? Which interpretations may be most helpful for this audience to hear? What can Christians say about the death of Jesus that might help trauma survivors experience love and grace in the midst of their suffering?

RETHINKING THE DEATH OF JESUS

One place to begin developing an interpretation of the cross that may speak to some trauma survivors is with the theme of divine solidarity.[22] On this view, Jesus enters, in his life and ministry, into the situation of the oppressed and struggles with them against the injustices they face. This life lived in opposition to injustice ultimately leads him to his death on the cross. Jesus' sufferings, however, are not just his own; they are also the sufferings of all others, which he shares with them. Moreover, since God was in Jesus, the cross is not just Jesus' but also God's act of solidarity with the oppressed. On the cross, Jesus identifies God with victims of innocent suffering. While this suffering cannot be justified, the fact that God embraces it shows the lengths to which God goes to overcome human social alienation and estrangement. God does not remain aloof from human suffering but enters into this suffering, sharing the pain it causes.[23]

For some trauma survivors, this view of the cross as an act of divine solidarity may function as a source of healing by enabling them to see their reality in Jesus' sufferings; their trauma is now not only theirs but also his. This identification of Jesus' sufferings with the survivor's can prove helpful in overcoming their isolation and alienation, mitigating their pain. As Terrell observes, speaking from her own experience with violence as well as from her analysis of the cross in African American Christian traditions, some survivors find redemptive value in the cross by seeing it as "a supreme reminder of God's *with-us-ness* (that is, of God's decision to be *at-one* with us; or, better said, of the fact that we are already *at-one*)."[24]

In the church, however, the solidarity or "with-ness" that people experience must include not only the presence of Jesus but also the loving support of the community. This support constitutes an important part of what it means for the church to shape its life around the narratives of Jesus' life, death, and resurrection. When people in the church participate in Jesus' story through their practices, they also participate in each other's stories, which are all held within the larger narratives of Jesus. Concretely, this participation in each other's stories can take place through aspects of the church's life and worship, such as times of sharing of joys and concerns and small group discussions, prayers, and meditations. The witnessing function of the church requires that its members embody such openness to each other's pain; as a community that commits itself to bear witness to the suffering of the world, the church is called to be a fellowship of mutual openness and support. For some traumatized persons, the knowledge that the community (as well as God) is with them in their pain can further take away trauma's power to alienate and give them a larger, shared narrative into which their stories can be placed, a framework that holds together the fragments of traumatic memory.

While the solidarity of the Christian community may assist some survivors, it would make just a small contribution to their healing if it entailed merely empathy and emotional support. As Joanne Carlson Brown and Rebecca Parker observe, the idea that Jesus and the community participate in their suffering can give survivors psychological comfort, but it does not change the social conditions that led to their traumas.[25] Solidarity, in this limited sense of the term, makes suffering more bearable but does not take the suffering away. Especially in situations in which the traumas are repeated and ongoing, we need a broader view of solidarity that moves beyond sympathetic companionship to include actions that concretely address the conditions of violence. For example, in the case of an abuse victim who faces violence at home, the church's solidarity would entail not only listening to his story but also helping him find ways to survive and resist the violence. Similarly, for the flood survivor who has lost her home, solidarity would include providing her with a place to stay and material resources.

This understanding of solidarity can have its roots in the biblical narratives of Jesus. As Yoder observes, the gospels indicate that Jesus' ministry of creating a new human community involved transforming the status quo so that those who suffer could live life more abundantly. This challenge to the powers ultimately led to his death, as he refused to acquiesce to the powers and instead continued to embody an alternative way that denied their attempt to make him over into their own image.[26] By emphasizing that Jesus' death resulted from his resistance to the powers and not from submission to them, Christians underscore that the cross does not valorize human suffering. To claim that God identifies with those who suffer does not encourage their victimization; as Yoder contends, suffering is not the goal of the Christian life (and Christians thus do not need to be traumatized to experience the cross as meaningful). Instead of demanding that Christians seek victimization, the biblical narratives acknowledge human suffering and, at the same time, issue a call to a new life of resistance and transformation.

MEMORY AND THE CROSS

While the discussion of divine (and human) solidarity offers one resource for understanding how the symbol of the cross might facilitate recovery from trauma, this interpretation of the cross goes only so far in developing a theological description of healing. The concept of solidarity sheds light on how the survivor's alienation can be mitigated; however, healing from trauma involves much more than this. Recall that another common effect of trauma is the recirculation of painful memories in the survivors' bodies and minds, which can alienate them from themselves as well as from their communities. For some survivors, intrusive memories fracture their "old" selves over time, such that their healing must involve the creation of a "new" self that integrates the memories of the trauma and thereby lessens their power to retraumatize. From a theological perspective, this account of trauma and memory raises the questions: Can the cross help to facilitate not only the overcoming of social alienation but also the retrieval and transformation of traumatic memories? Can the survivors' integration of their story into communal narratives that tell of Jesus' death transform the memories of trauma held within their bodies and minds? Or would the symbol of the cross reinvoke these memories in ways that retraumatize the survivor?

As noted above, some feminist and womanist theologians do worry that for trauma survivors the symbol of the cross will evoke traumatic memories that are simply overwhelming. In an article entitled "Trauma and Grace," Serene Jones relates the emblematic story of one survivor in the church who became terrified during the celebration of the Eucharist when the minister evoked the image of Jesus' broken body and blood. For this woman, the image of violence in the church's liturgy brought to mind memories of her own abuse, making her feel as though she were once again reliving the trauma.[27] As trauma scholars observe, painful traumatic memories often surface when survivors confront cues in their environments—even seemingly insignificant ones—that remind them of their traumas. Given that the cross symbolizes a violent event of torture, it is not surprising that it could sometimes function in this way.

While the cross may represent for some individuals a symbol of terror that plays upon their traumatic experiences, it may contribute for others to the healing of traumatic memory by facilitating the narrative reconstruction of their traumas. Recall the claim of some trauma theorists that part of what makes it possible for people to remember and narrate their traumatic experiences is to see these experiences symbolized in ways that are both similar to and different from their own stories. The similarity between the images of trauma and the survivor's own experience activates the traumatic memory and enables him or her to confront it; the difference allows the traumatic structure of the memory to be transformed.[28] As van der Kolk and his colleagues observe, the most critical difference in transforming traumatic memories is the setting in which survivors confront the images of their traumas.[29] By interacting with these images in a safe setting, they can begin to modify the intense emotions the traumas evoke and alter their interpretations of these events. In the church, when survivors find dimensions of their own stories in the narratives of Jesus—when they see similarities between his story and theirs—they may recall (and perhaps tell the story of) their own traumas.[30] Only now they may remember and narrate these stories in a different context: the context of a supportive community.[31]

How, precisely, might this narration of one's trauma in Christian community contribute to the healing process? One theory suggests that by narrating their traumas to others within a supportive community, survivors externalize their stories and then reinternalize them, along with the compassionate responses of the listeners.[32] This internalization of the listeners' responses may change how they remember their traumas in multiple ways. For example, it may enable them to see how they exercised their own agency, the reasons they did not deserve what happened to them, and their own strengths that enabled them to survive. In addition, the compassionate responses also may help them to remember their traumas not as events they endure alone but as ones they share with others. In the church, then, when people form relationships of solidarity and trust that enable testimony and witnessing, survivors may narrate their traumas in a way that alters the traumatic character of the memories. Note, however, that this narration does not necessarily involve the verbal telling of the trauma narratives. Through their participation in the church's practices, people can "tell" or narrate their stories by placing them within the communal narratives that the church shares, the ongoing narratives of Jesus.

On its own, the logic of solidarity remains inadequate to explain how the symbol of the cross might contribute to the transformation of traumatic memory. Only the logic of solidarity and difference together can accomplish this. Whereas trauma theorists focus on the differences in the social contexts in which the survivor interacts with images of trauma—the differences between a supportive and non-supportive context—we must explore as well the theological distinctions between Jesus' trauma and the survivors' own experiences. The content of these narratives and the ways they are interpreted, not just the social context in which they are encountered, helps to determine whether interaction with the gospel narratives of the crucifixion cultivates healing for trauma survivors.

Two theological differences between the sufferings of Jesus and those of trauma survivors in the church are especially important. First, unlike many trauma survivors who had no choice to avoid the violence they faced, Jesus' sufferings on the cross resulted from a way of life that he voluntarily chose. This does not mean that Jesus sought suffering for its own sake or that he elected to suffer and die a painful death, but rather that he freely chose to live a life of social nonconformity in relation to the powers, a life that resulted in the cross. In his ministry, Jesus consciously embodied a sociopolitical-ethical stance of nonviolent resistance to injustice in the world. This stance led to his confrontation with the ruling authorities and, ultimately, to his death.[33]

On one level, stressing the voluntary character of Jesus' sufferings risks recapitulating the notion that people must choose to suffer to be like him (and thus worthy in God's eyes). To guard against this interpretation, it is important to emphasize that the sufferings Jesus elected to endure did not come from either abuse or a random violent event but from his active opposition to injustice. Being like Jesus, then, entails choosing to oppose violence through nonviolent means. When this point is underscored, the emphasis on the voluntary character of his sufferings may remind survivors that their own traumas resulted not from their choices but from the choices of others. This may help them to see that they are not responsible for these harms, though they are responsible for their healing and for breaking the cycle of violence.[34] When understood in this way, the narratives of Jesus' life and death may enable survivors to see their traumas as unjust while challenging them to resist the ongoing effects of this harm.

The second important difference that distinguishes Jesus' sufferings from trauma survivors' is that within the Christian traditions, the former are linked with the promise of transformation and new life for the world. Recall Yoder's assertion that the cross is the kingdom come, an event in which Jesus triumphs over the powers and principalities by refusing to conform to their violent ways. In so doing, he inaugurates the new aeon, creating a new human community that embodies an alternative, nonviolent way of being in the world. As Christians locate their own stories in the context of this narrative of new possibility, they may come to know that their lives are now placed within a framework that includes not only a story of traumatic violence but also the promise of redemption and new life. Moreover, participating in the church may already place one in a context in which this promise can be experienced, though not to its fullest.

The cross, as the convergence of the old and new aeons, can thus be a symbol that heals as well as one that terrifies. It is the inbreaking of the kingdom as well as an event of traumatic violence. In the context of church practices, images of the cross can both evoke traumatic memories and speak a word of hope. In its multivocality, the cross tells not just of an event of torture but also of Jesus' compassion for the victims (and the perpetrators) of suffering.[35] In suffering on the cross, Jesus makes it clear that victims do not suffer alone. In refusing to respond to his enemies with sheer force, he breaks the link between the self as site of violence and the self as agent of violence. Declining to be made over into the violent image of the powers, he triumphs over them and thereby frees others to live apart from their control. Through the communal enactment of his story, Christians embody this new life that he makes possible and thereby integrate themselves into his ongoing narrative, a narrative that neither effaces nor valorizes their pain but places it in the context of both God's and the community's loving presence with them.

THE RESURRECTION OF JESUS

This promise of new life, however, becomes evident only when considering the meaning of the resurrection in relation to the crucifixion. Recall that for Yoder, Jesus' resurrection shows that God's redeeming power is stronger than the power of evil and that God, through the work of Jesus, has triumphed over the powers. Moreover, Yoder argues that God's redeeming power is manifest not only through Jesus' resurrection in the past but also in the present. God's Spirit is at work in the world, and through this Spirit, human beings can have present-day experiences of healing and transformation that will have a future consummation. Here, he draws on the logic of solidarity but extends it to include the resurrection as well as the cross. Just as Jesus identifies with those who suffer, so do they participate in his resurrection: "we can talk about the resurrection of Christ as somehow drawing us along in a promised (future) resurrection."[36]

In their life and worship, Christians remember this promised future of resurrection and new life in many ways. For example, on Sunday mornings church members sing hymns and listen to sermons which proclaim that Christ has risen from the dead. As noted above, Christians also often speak of the ritual of baptism as a "dying and rising" with Christ. In addition, many churches repeat the familiar refrain when they celebrate the eucharist: "Christ has died, Christ has risen, Christ will come again." As Christians enact the story of Jesus through their life and worship, they recall not only the past of his (and their own) suffering, but also a promised future of restoration and transformation.

When they place their traumas into this larger narrative context that includes the resurrection of Jesus as well as his life and death, survivors do not obliterate or deny their personal stories but set these stories in a new framework, one that transforms their meaning and takes away their gripping or totalizing force. In the church, individuals integrate their stories into a shared narrative that both recognizes the woundedness of humanity and proclaims that this woundedness is being redeemed. This proclamation that the redemption of their traumas has begun (and will have a future consummation) may give traumatized persons a sense of renewal in the midst of their despair, a hope that yet acknowledges the unpredictability of life and the reality of their pain. As trauma theorists note, this recontextualization of the trauma—its integration into a larger, communal narrative that tempers fear and disillusionment with hope—is necessary for the traumas to lose their totalizing power. Once recontextualized, the survivors' traumatic experiences cease to dominate their lives.

The recontextualization of the survivors' stories in the narratives of Jesus does not, however, lead to an easy resolution of their traumas. The resurrection does not provide the "answer" to the crucifixion, nor does it offer survivors a comforting hope that simply eliminates their fear and despair. As trauma theorists observe, healing from trauma is never easy. Thus, while the resurrection may provide a much-needed word of hope for some survivors, it does not simply take away their suffering.

Moreover, the resurrection itself issues a challenge that can profoundly unsettle some persons: It calls them to choose life, to refuse to stay with crucifixion. For many trauma survivors, this choice for life involves seeking to heal from their traumas, a choice that can prove difficult insofar as it requires them to face the stories of their lives and confront the overwhelming past. Paradoxically, this choice for life that the resurrection both enables and demands can bring additional pain; healing involves more suffering precisely because it requires dealing with painful memories and emotions. As trauma theorists note, the choice for life is an ongoing process. Often, people move on to the next stage of healing only to find that they later must return to issues they have already addressed. From a theological perspective, this pattern of alternating between experiencing pain and moving forward in the healing process is represented by the dialectical relationship between the cross and resurrection. The resurrection does not cancel out the cross, but neither does the cross deny the truth of the resurrection.

REDEMPTION IN TRAUMA STUDIES AND CHRISTIAN THEOLOGY

The theological reflections offered so far in this chapter have focused on ways in which the church's communal enactment of the gospel narratives might cultivate healing from trauma. For this analysis, I have taken as my starting place several points on which trauma studies and Christian theology share some basic agreement. Both disciplines consider narrative central to the formation of the "self," both describe ways in which individuals contextualize their stories within a broader narrative, and both see the self's transformation through this contextualization as an ongoing process. In the course of exploring these convergences and their usefulness for theologically understanding recovery from trauma, a few differences between trauma theory and theology surfaced as well. For example, the latter focuses on shared, communal narratives while the former primarily speaks of individual narratives. Moreover, the theological framework that I have outlined explores the process of enacting a narrative, whereas traditional trauma paradigms concentrate on the action of verbally telling one's narrative.

An obvious difference that I have not yet explicitly considered now warrants attention: the divergent views of "redemption" that one finds in these two disciplines. For many trauma theorists, a trauma is "redeemed" when survivors find meaning in its aftermath, not by being glad the traumas happened or agreeing that they served a larger purpose such as fulfilling God's plan, but by finding that some good has come out of the recovery process, even though the traumas themselves were not good.[37] Recall, for instance, that survivors may find they have become a stronger person or that they can use their experiences to help others. Herman explains, "While there is no way to compensate for an atrocity, there is a way to transcend it, by making it a gift to others. The trauma is redeemed only when it becomes the source of a survivor mission."[38]

The Christian traditions offer a more complex view of redemption. From a Christian theological perspective, the reality of God's redemption means that while our losses are never erased, God promises us a future in which we are no longer trapped in our brokenness and in which our injuries are healed, a future in which life, love, and relationships are reconstructed.[39] The gospels depict this dimension of redemption through the eschatological image of the wounded Christ who appears to his disciples in transfigured form.[40] In some ways, this image resonates with trauma scholars' views of healing: The wounds remain but are transformed. In the Christian traditions, however, this transformation entails not only the healing of one's broken spirit but also the resurrection of one's body. Christians ground this belief that bodies are resurrected in the conviction that the resurrection of Jesus by God's Spirit functions as a sign of what will happen to all people in the fulfillment of God's kingdom. Just as the resurrected Jesus is restored but still recognizable as himself, so will we be both transformed and the same.

Unlike secular views of redemption, theological accounts understand redemption as the work of God, either wholly apart from or in concert with human activity. According to the Christian traditions, redemption is the work God does through Jesus and the Spirit. Jesus redeems humanity in his life, death, and resurrection by achieving solidarity with us in our suffering, by atoning for our sins, and by destroying death and all that would harm us. The Spirit continues to empower people by giving the gift of new life that renews and supports us. Thus, whereas trauma scholars see redemption as an internal, psychological process in which the individual, with the support of others, finds meaning in his or her own life and in the world, Christian theology claims that redemption involves God giving meaning to the world through the work of Jesus and the Spirit. This emphasis on God's work suggests that Christians can find healing, in part, by looking outside themselves to their communal narratives that describe God's redemptive activity. Note, however, that a theological framework does not say that God's agency overwhelms or operates in place of human agency, but rather that God is the ground, support, and goal of human agency. Thus, in the church trauma survivors participate in their own healing but are empowered to do so by something larger than themselves: God's grace as expressed through the Christian community.

In Christian theology, however, God's redeeming power extends beyond the human community. Whereas trauma theory focuses on the redemption of the individual's life, many Christian traditions apply their belief in God's transformative power to the world as well. From this perspective, redemption involves the promise of a communal future, the kingdom of God, in which all of creation enjoys communion with God and with each other. In speaking of God's kingdom, Christians point to a future they believe Jesus inaugurated in his life, death, and resurrection, a future that will be consummated when the whole creation is transformed through the fulfillment and completion of God's creative and redemptive work. As this emphasis on God's work makes clear, Christians maintain that the kingdom does not grow out of this world; it is not developed through human efforts and does not emerge from the potentialities of the present.[41] Rather, it is a new thing that comes as a gift from God, gathering up what is and transforming it.[42]

When will this transformation take place? On the one hand, Christian theology speaks of God's kingdom as a future reality. On the other hand, it maintains that the present contains anticipations of this future. Redemption is not simply for a later time; it has begun. God's redemptive reality thus has an already/not yet character: Human beings have present-day experiences of transformation and the promise that this transformation will have a future consummation. As discussed in chapter 1, Yoder argues that the church represents one place people would ideally experience a foretaste of this future. As a community that confesses faith in Jesus, the church is called to live as the new humanity he inaugurated, the first fruits of God's redemptive reality. It is called to hold up signs of God's kingdom, though these signs are never unbroken and unambiguous.[43]

When the Christian community holds up these signs by performing the narratives of Jesus, it can help to facilitate the reconstruction of the identities of those who constitute the church. For some trauma survivors, this reconstruction of their identities may begin to transform some of the trauma's effects: As they integrate themselves into the narratives of Jesus, survivors may locate their own traumas within a broader framework, overcome some of their isolation and alienation, and temper their fear and disillusionment with a sense of hope. I have suggested that the narratives which the church performs can facilitate this transformation by acknowledging (but not valorizing) the reality of trauma and framing this reality within a redemptive story that refuses to offer simplistic solutions that trivialize the survivor's pain. Traumatized persons who participate in the church's performance of these narratives may find that while the trauma continues to remain integral to their identities, its totalizing force is now challenged by the alternative vision of God's redemptive reality.

The creation of a context in which traumatized persons can experience healing constitutes an integral part of Christian nonviolence and thus a crucial dimension of what it means to "be the church." Like the enactment of voluntary, egalitarian, and witnessing relationships, the performance of the biblical narratives constitutes an important part of the church's everyday life as a community called to exist as the new social humanity Jesus created. Through its life and worship, the church embodies and internalizes the narratives of Jesus, which tell of trauma and resistance, violence and redemption.

Moving beyond ecclesial relations and the enactment of a communal narrative, I now turn in the final chapter to a third possible resource for healing that Christian communities may offer simply by "being the church": the formation of an eschatological community that participates in the transformation of the world. By bringing this dimension of the life to which the church is called into conversation with the third phase of recovery from trauma, I take the theological analysis of healing offered here one step further. This, in turn, leads to a new understanding of Christian nonviolence.

NOTES

1. Jane Miller [pseudo.], conversation with the author, New Haven, CT, July 7, 2003.

2. For example, see Delores Williams, *Sisters in the Wilderness: The Challenge of Womanist God-Talk* (Maryknoll, NY: Orbis Books, 1993); Joanne Carlson Brown and Rebecca Parker, "For God So Loved the World?" in *Christianity, Patriarchy, and Abuse: A Feminist Critique*, eds. Joanne Carlson Brown and Carole R. Bohn (New York: Pilgrim Press, 1989), 1–30; Rita Nakashima Brock and Rebecca Parker, *Proverbs of Ashes: Violence, Redemptive Suffering, and the Search for What Saves Us* (Boston: Beacon Press, 2001).

3. See Donna Kane, Sharon E. Cheston, and Joanne Greer, "Perceptions of God by Survivors of Childhood Sexual Abuse: An Exploratory Study in an Underresearched Area," 235.

4. For a helpful account of the role of narrative in Yoder's work and his relationship to narrative theology, see Chris Huebner, "Mennonites and Narrative Theology: The Case of John Howard Yoder," *The Conrad Grebel Review*, 16 (1998): 15–38.

5. Harry Huebner, cited in Chris Huebner, "Mennonites and Narrative Theology," 34.

6. Huebner, "Mennonites and Narrative Theology," 29. On the performative dimension of Christian practices, see also Shannon Craigo-Snell, "Command Performance: Rethinking Performance Interpretation in the Context of Divine Discourse," *Modern Theology* 16 no. 4 (October 2000): 475–94.

7. Yoder, *Body Politics.*, ix.

8. Yoder, *Body Politics*, 72–73.

9. This notion that Christians become "characters" who are "crafted" through their communal enactment of the biblical texts comes from Shannon Craigo-Snell's analysis of Christian practices as embodied performances in "Command Performance," 480.

10. Yoder, *Body Politics*, 73.

11. Dori Laub, "Bearing Witness," 69.

12. Laub, "Bearing Witness," 69.

13. See Laub, "Bearing Witness" and "An Event Without Witness."

14. Flora Keshgegian also observes that the cross of Jesus represents a traumatic event. She argues that just as healing from trauma involves connecting one's own story to a bigger narrative in which trauma does not dominate, so must the Christian community "decenter" the crucifixion and tell the story of Jesus in a way that does not allow his death to overwhelm the rest of the narrative. Keshgegian argues, "The crucifixion by itself is not effective for redemption; it can only provide a partial message of salvation" (*Redeeming Memories,* 174). In another place, however, she suggests that the cross has no salvific significance: "The cross is not redeemable. It is not redemptive. The cross is horrible and tragic. It must be mourned and remembered" (196). As noted above, I agree with Keshgegian's former claim that the cross does have salvific significance, when taken in the broader context of Jesus' life and resurrection. The Christian traditions, beginning with the canonical gospels, contain rich resources for holding together these different aspects of Jesus' life without allowing one to dominate; Yoder's work represents a good example.

15. The term "mimetic reproductions of violence" has two different meanings. First, it refers to the way in which interpretations of the cross that focus on Jesus' sacrifice and suffering can be used to prevent people from resisting structural and interpersonal violence (see Joanne Carlson Brown and Rebecca Parker, "For God So Loved the World?" and Delores Williams, *Sisters in the Wilderness*). Second, it denotes how the cross can mimetically reproduce violence by functioning as a symbol of terror that evokes traumatic flashbacks and intrusive memories. I address this issue below.

16. Williams, *Sisters in the Wilderness,* 165.

17. Terrell, *Power in the Blood?: The Cross in the African American Experience* (Maryknoll, NY: Orbis Books, 1998), 34.

18. Terrell, *Power in the Blood?* 125.

19. Yoder, *Politics of Jesus,* 238.

20. Terrell, *Power in the Blood?* 125.

21. Flora Keshgegian, *Redeeming Memories,* 174.

22. One can interpret the cross in other ways that might resonate with non-traumatized persons as well. Moreover, this understanding of the cross as an event in which God acts in solidarity with those who suffer may prove meaningful for some persons who are not traumatized as well as those who are. As discussed in chapter 2, some who have not endured traumas may experience, to a lesser degree, trauma-like symptoms such as alienation, anxiety, and despair.

23. This interpretation draws on the work of Jürgen Moltmann, *The Crucified God: The Cross of Christ as the Foundation and Criticism of Christian Theology,* trans. by R. A. Wilson and John Bowden (Minneapolis: Fortress Press, 1993). For a critique of the notion of the suffering God, see Johann M. Vento, "Violence, Trauma, and Resistance: A Feminist Appraisal of Metz's Mysticism of Suffering Unto God," *Horizons* 29: 1 (Spring 2002): 7–22.

24. Terrell, *Power in the Blood?* 125.

25. Brown and Parker, "For God So Loved the World?," 17.

26. See Yoder, *The Politics of Jesus*, ch. 8.

27. Jones, "Trauma and Grace," in *Reflections*, Yale Divinity School (Winter 2004): 11. Here, we see the potential harmful effects of emphasizing that the cross is about divine solidarity. If survivors are unable to see the difference between themselves and Jesus, then images of Jesus' suffering may invoke their traumatic memories rather than help them to overcome their sense of social alienation and isolation.

28. Van der Kolk, McFarlane, and van der Hart, "A General Approach to Treatment," 430.

29. Van der Kolk, McFarlane, and van der Hart, "A General Approach to Treatment," 431.

30. Cynthia Crysdale makes a similar point. She writes, "By identifying with Jesus the Crucified, one is able to name one's own victimization, to face the wounds that have hampered one's full human flourishing." *Embracing Travail: Retrieving the Cross Today* (New York: Continuum, 1999), 10.

31. This part of the healing process thus depends on both divine and human solidarity: the survivor's experiencing Jesus' solidarity with them and the community's offer of support.

32. See Aaron Mishara's analysis of healing in his article "Narrative and Psychotherapy—the Phenomenology of Healing," 180–95.

33. See Yoder, *The Politics of Jesus*, ch. 8.

34. Herman, *Trauma and Recovery*, 192.

35. On the multivocality of symbols, see Victor Turner, "Social Dramas and Ritual Metaphors," *Dramas, Fields, and Metaphors: Symbolic Action in Human Society* (New York: Cornell University Press, Inc., 1974), 55.

36. John Howard Yoder, *Preface to Theology: Christology and Theological Method* (Grand Rapids: Eerdmans, 2002), 105.

37. Brison, *Aftermath*, 20.

38. Herman, *Trauma and Recovery*, 207.

39. Brokenness here includes the sins we commit as well as those we suffer.

40. See John 20:19ff.

41. See Jürgen Moltmann, *Theology of Hope: On the Ground and the Implications of Christian Eschatology* (New York: Harper & Row, 1967).

42. See Moltmann, *Theology of Hope*.

43. Yoder, "The Spirit of God and the Politics of Men," in *For the Nations*, 234.

6

Enacting an Eschatological Identity

While reflecting on the ways her recovery process has transformed her life, one abuse survivor remarked, "I don't live stuck in the past anymore. I can now see that the world has many positive possibilities, and they are open to me."[1] In describing this change, she points to a dimension of healing that trauma theorists commonly identify as central to the third phase of recovery: the retemporalization of the traumatized person. Once survivors have given their traumas temporal and spatial location by placing them in a narrative framework, they can themselves experience a different orientation toward time. They can stop being consumed by the past and, in turn, fully engage the present by deepening their life-giving relationships, developing plans for their future, and putting these plans into action. In this chapter I theologically reflect on this final stage of healing to illuminate a third way the church may enable recovery just by "being the church."

Yoder's view of the church as an eschatological community provides the basis for these reflections. Recall that for Yoder, an integral part of what it means for the church to be the church is to communally enact a life of faithful discipleship and thereby take part in the new (but not fully realized) order, or eschaton, ushered in by Jesus. In articulating this vision of Christian community, Yoder points to an overlapping of times that both resonates with and differs from the one that trauma theorists describe. Trauma theorists claim that for many traumatized persons, the past arrests the present as traumatic memories and emotions continually resurface against their will. By contrast, Yoder contends that the future—the future of God's kingdom—moves into the present with the life, death, and resurrection of Jesus and becomes manifest in the church as it conforms to his way of life.[2] From the perspective of trauma studies, this view of Christian community raises the questions: How might it affect traumatized persons to participate in a community that lives as a site of this "eschatological overlapping"? Can the overlapping of times that Yoder points to help foster their retemporalization? What resources for recovery can it offer to trauma survivors, and what problems might it pose?

In this chapter I argue that the church, as an eschatological community, may contribute to the retemporalization of trauma survivors by offering them an opportunity to claim (and be claimed by) a communal future that differs from their traumatic past. As the words of the survivor quoted above indicate, coming to claim or "own" a hopeful vision for the future represents a key part of the final phase of healing. In the first phase survivors establish the supportive relationships that provide a necessary context for developing a new vision of oneself, others, and the world. In the second phase, survivors can, with the help of this support, place their traumas within a broader narrative that enables them to see the world's life-giving possibilities. In the third phase, survivors then come to view these possibilities as open to themselves.

In the church, some trauma survivors may develop and claim a hopeful vision for their own futures by participating in the communal enactment of the narratives of Jesus. As they take part in the church's life and worship, they may come to see their futures as included in the open and abundant communal future that the biblical narratives proclaim and that the church realizes, albeit in a markedly incomplete way. Survivors may receive meaning and identity, therefore, not only from their individual past and present but also from the future of God's redemptive reality as it impinges on the present. This reality deepens their sense that God's love as manifest through the community will enable them to flourish and resist being overwhelmed by the brokenness of the world. And this, in turn, may give traumatized persons the motivation and power to engage in what trauma theorists call a "survivor mission" and act as agents of transformation in the world.

The church does not, however, assist all traumatized persons with this part of the healing process. As discussed previously, for some traumatized persons, the experience of trauma raises such troubling theological questions that they simply cannot look to religious communities as a possible resource for healing. Unable to find a satisfactory explanation for how God could allow such horrible things to happen, they turn elsewhere for support. Some others who do look to the church encounter another obstacle: to construct and claim an empowering vision for the future entails imagining how what is to come may differ from the past; however, as noted in chapter 2, survivors sometimes experience a constricted imagination that makes it difficult to conceive of a future which does not repeat the harmful patterns of the past.[3] In the pages ahead, I suggest one way that the church, just by "being the church," can address this difficulty: simply by living as a foretaste of the new future Jesus proclaimed. In doing so, the church creates a context in which survivors experience an alternative to their traumatic past. This experience, in turn, may expand their capacity to imagine a broader range of possibilities.

As these introductory remarks indicate, chapters 5 and 6 of this book are interrelated. My reflections in these chapters overlap because of an important difference that distinguishes my theological analysis of healing from the theoretical reflections that many trauma theorists offer. When trauma theorists describe the healing process, they often identify integrating the trauma into a broader narrative as central to phase two and claiming a positive vision for the future as part of phase three. The theological account of healing that I develop understands these two aspects of recovery as intertwined: Christians integrate their traumas into a shared narrative that itself contains a hopeful vision for the future, and they come to own this vision partly by integrating themselves into the narrative through the community's practice of it. While it thus remains impossible to separate completely the material contained in these two chapters, the following analysis does deepen the reflections previously offered. This "deepening" leads to a reconceptualization of Christian nonviolence that the insights of trauma theory require—one that addresses the reality of internalized, traumatic violence. By exploring this new understanding of nonviolence, we can better grasp how selves and communities can become not only sites of violence, but also sites of grace.

OWNING THE NARRATIVES OF JESUS

In reflecting on her childhood experiences of the church, one trauma survivor recalls a day when her pastor showed his congregation an illustration of children gathered around Jesus' feet. Intended to represent Jesus' love for children, the picture evoked in this survivor instead a profound sense of alienation. "I felt as though I did not belong in the picture," she remarked. "Everyone else was welcome at Jesus' feet, but I was somehow not included."[4] Years later this picture she had seen as a child became to her an image of hope. In describing her long process of healing she stated, "When I now think of what it means to heal, I think of being held in the lap of God."[5]

Her comment identifies an important transition in her recovery process from encountering an alternative narrative that offers a word of hope to internalizing or coming to own this narrative. As the survivor's words indicate, it is one thing to hear the story of Jesus and another to feel included within it. For some survivors, claiming such an alternative narrative as their own—coming to see that the story gives expression to their reality and that they deserve to participate in the good news it proclaims—constitutes an essential part of retemporalization. When they not only integrate their traumas into a broader, redemptive framework but also deeply internalize the messages of hope this framework contains, survivors can be finally freed from the past, engage the present, and anticipate the future. In chapter 5 I began to explore how the church might contribute to this dimension of healing by offering a narrative that both recognizes trauma and promises redemption, and by creating a context in which people enact this narrative through the community's social practices.

This understanding of how trauma survivors may claim or internalize this narrative—and a specific challenge they may face in doing so—deepens if we return to the subject of memory and integrate into it the critical component of imagination.[6] As Kirmayer observes, there exists a fundamental connection between "memory and imagination, retelling and re-creating the self."[7] This connection may not appear obvious at first. According to Majorie Procter-Smith, we often think of memory and imagination as mutually exclusive. We understand memory as the recollection of facts, and imagination as "flights of fancy unfettered by anything so mundane as historical events."[8]

Memory and imagination, however, are connected in at least two ways. First, our memories of the past are shaped by our imagination. As Kirmayer observes, "Memory is anything but a photographic record of experience; it is a roadway full of potholes, badly in need of repair, worked on day and night by revisionist crews."[9] When we remember, we "fill in the gaps" in our memories and interpret the significance of what we recall. In so doing, we exercise one important dimension of imagination: the capacity to develop a particular way of seeing reality, of making sense of the world around us.[10] For survivors to construct narratives of their traumas—to re-remember their memories—in a way that reinterprets their significance, then, is itself an imaginative act. I have argued that the church may help survivors to re-imagine their traumatic memories precisely by providing a broader narrative into which these memories can be incorporated, a framework that contains an event of trauma contextualized within a larger story of God's love and compassion. When they place their own stories within this broader narrative, trauma survivors may come to re-vision their traumatic experiences as ones that are shared by God (and a community) and included within God's redemptive reality.

A second connection between memory and imagination makes the role of imagination in the healing process more complex. Not only are our memories shaped by our imagination, but our imaginative visions of the future also are funded by memory. On the one hand, imagining a future that is different from the past requires us to transcend the knowledge we have gained from our past and present experiences; imagination, in this sense, has a prophetic function. On the other hand, this vision of the future does not remain entirely divorced from our memory. As theologian Trevor Hart explains, human beings cannot imagine things that have no basis in our knowledge of the past and present. We can only "modify the known" in such a way that the resulting vision differs significantly from our memories of past and present experiences.[11] Since even this modification draws on what we know of the world more broadly, imagination is always either overtly or subtly funded by memory.

For trauma survivors who experience constricted imagination, the task of creating a hopeful vision for the future may prove especially challenging. Recall that some survivors are consumed by intrusive thoughts about the past and thus remain unable to conceive of a future that is fundamentally different. When their memories of trauma continually intrude into the present, their imaginative visions of the future—to the extent that they can envision the future at all—are bleak indeed. This raises the questions: How could survivors whose "knowns" contain little that is positive grasp the hopeful vision that the church proclaims? How can they not only hear this vision but also concretely imagine it and see it as including themselves?

When their past "knowns" do not provide much basis for imagining and claiming the hopeful vision that the church proclaims, Christians may still come to own this vision precisely by experiencing it in the present in small ways. Recall that for Yoder, the eschatological vision of the church is not mere fantasy but something the church embodies and expresses now, albeit in broken form. If the identities of the church and its members are formed by biblical narratives that tell of kindness and grace, justice and mercy, and love and compassion, then survivors in the church may have their "knowns" expanded to include hopeful elements. As they not only hear stories about goodness but also take part in a community that embodies voluntary and egalitarian relationships and that practices traditions which manifest God's grace, survivors may find that all this becomes part of their knowns that they can then imaginatively modify.

This expansion of their knowns may make it possible for some survivors to integrate into their identities the eschatological vision that the church proclaims. Through their participation in the community's life and worship, Christians place themselves within an ongoing story that "remembers" the future as well as the past.[12] As they perform the story of Jesus, they remember that God's promise to remain faithful to them extends beyond the present into the future. This memory of God's future faithfulness becomes constitutive of their identities, an integral part of who they are—a memory that shapes their understanding of themselves, others, and the world.

This integration, of course, is not something the church does on its own. Recall that for Yoder, Christian practices are the work of God, "in and with, through and under" what human beings do.[13] The eschatological vision that people receive in the church, therefore, comes to them in part through the work of the Spirit, who, as Hart contends, frees their imaginations and "opens up for [them] a new vision of God's promise" for the future and a new perspective on the world in the present.[14] This vision that the Christian community proclaims and strives to embody is thus, at its deepest level, a gift from God.

As God's gift, this eschatological vision has an external character: It comes from outside of what Christians know about the world, bringing something beyond their imaginations.[15] At the same time, this vision is not entirely removed from present-day realities. As the "already" and "not yet" character of Christian eschatology indicates, the future of God's redemptive reality has begun. Though the Christian community does not bring about this future, it can provide a context in which people experience anticipations of it by enacting relationships of peace, justice, and love. As Yoder observes, the church is called to do more than merely point to the vision of the future that helps ground its life and identity. It is also called to live as the first fruits of this vision by constituting an alternative community that exists as a foretaste of the kingdom of God.

This view of the church as a foretaste of the kingdom reveals a crucial difference between the retemporalization many trauma theorists describe and the theological retemporalization I am outlining here. Trauma scholars suggest that retemporalization involves freeing oneself from the past, engaging the present, and envisioning the future with hope. In contrast, a theological analysis suggests that retemporalization entails not only envisioning this future but also, to a certain degree, participating in it now. The retemporalization that may happen in the church is, therefore, an eschatological retemporalization: The Christian community not only engages the present and hopes for the future, it also embodies this future (though never in unbroken form). Through its creation of an alternative community that lives in faithful discipleship to Jesus, the church chooses to be claimed by, and to claim as its own, the communal future he inaugurated.

This understanding of eschatological retemporalization indicates that healing from trauma can take place, at least in part, through the communal construction of a new identity. In its life and worship, the church enacts a new *eschatological* identity, an identity shaped not only by the past and present but also by the future as it impinges on the present. In enacting this eschatological identity (or becoming an eschatological community), persons in the church do not gain a second identity that simply sits alongside the first, nor do they acquire a new identity that erases the old. Rather, the old remains but is being transformed into the new.

This view of identity formation in the church differs from the claim of many trauma theorists' that survivors can reconstruct their identities in supportive communities. Whereas trauma theorists generally explore how traumatized persons heal through the reconstitution of their individual identities, a Christian theological framework sheds light on how individuals also can heal through their participation in the formation of a communal identity. As Christians enact a new communal identity by performing the narratives of Jesus, the identities of those who constitute the church are reformed to include not only their individual memories of past and present, but also their memory of a communal past and eschatological future.

This communal enactment of a new identity does not merely reconstitute the self, but also makes the self new.[16] From a theological perspective, one can speak of identities being made new because, as Trevor Hart observes, Christian eschatology maintains that God's promised future brings a new thing in the transformation and renewal of all things.[17] This new thing that God brings through the Spirit does not obliterate the old. Rather, the "old" and the "new" overlap—not in the sense that the old gives rise to the new, but in the sense that the new has already entered into the old and begun to transform it into what it ultimately will be.[18] As an eschatological community that strives to live as a foretaste of God's kingdom, the church exists as a site of this overlapping. It is called to participate in the new while living in the middle of and in contradiction to the old.[19]

In Christian community, then, persons may heal from the effects of trauma through the narrative construction and communal enactment of a new identity and through participation in the still incomplete new aeon that Jesus inaugurated. While this participation in the new does not erase the marks of the old, it does transform these marks and place them within a broader context. In their eschatological witness to Jesus, people in the church locate their own stories within a larger narrative framework that not only recalls past harms but also proclaims God's promise of a communal future in which all flourish and are made whole. Through its enactment of Christ's story, the church takes part in this new life he makes possible and thereby enacts an eschatological identity: the identity of the risen one who yet embodies the wounds of crucifixion.

HEALING AND THE BODY

This discussion of how Christians construct an eschatological identity points to an issue that trauma scholars often identify: the role of the body in healing from trauma. I have emphasized that the church's practices represent a central means through which Christians come to claim as their own a vision of an abundant future; and practices are, at a most basic level, embodied, communal performances.[20] In the church, people come to know God and claim Jesus' story by speaking not only with their mouths and voices but also with their whole bodies. For example, Christians stand and kneel in worship, wash each other's feet, and immerse people in water. They exchange a "kiss of peace," prepare food together, and consume bread and wine. In the Christian traditions, faith is not just something one says but also something one does. As Stephanie Paulsell observes, "Jesus' command that we love our neighbor as we love ourselves makes it clear that our faith has everything to do with how we live as embodied people."[21]

A central assumption of my argument is that embodied performances enable a more complete integration into the church's communal narratives than would mere verbal proclamation. By placing their whole selves into the narratives of Jesus, Christians come to know and to be formed by these stories in a deeper way. While they may know something of God's love when they hear that God cares for them, Christians know more fully what this means when they experience God's love through their relationships with others. Similarly, while some may believe that God suffers with them because others tell them this is so, they experience God's presence more deeply when they participate in a community that embodies Jesus' caring for outcasts and those who are injured.

In Christian community, healing thus involves the social as well as the individual body. Theologians speak of the church as a social body not just because it is partially comprised of individual bodies, but also because it involves the coordination of shared activities among people who work together and care for each other. As a social body, the church can participate in the healing of individual bodies through practices that "honor the body."[22] For example, Christians honor the body when they help people in need find shelter and care for the sick. They also honor the body through their practices that involve the use of touch in loving ways, such as foot washing and passing the peace. As Paulsell observes, such practices affirm that bodies deserve care and blessing, and they bring to mind the vulnerability of the body and the many injured bodies in the church and around the world. As Christians attend to the body, they are reminded of bodies that experience abuse, war, and illness.[23] Their remembrance of these bodies helps constitute them into a community in which each person cares for the bodies of others.

From a theological perspective, the image of the church as a social body offers a way to conceptualize the relational dimension of forming a new identity. Recall that trauma theorists often claim that individual bodies which experience trauma's ongoing effects can recover only in the context of healthy relationships. Christian theology portrays the church as ideally a community that constructs such relationships—relationships in which the community as a whole cares for individual "members" in need. Theologically, however, this image goes one step further to suggest not only that the healing of individual bodies is relational but also that the body itself is relational. The body of Christ image depicts the church as a mutually interdependent social organism in which each member is both unique and an important contributor to the whole. This view of the church suggests that Christians cannot speak of the wholeness of individual bodies—whether they have directly sustained traumatic injuries or not—apart from their participation in the social body. In Christian community, individual bodies are integrated or whole only when they both receive care from others and take part in giving such care.

My reflections on trauma and healing over the last three chapters have identified different dimensions of the relation between individual and social bodies. They have focused on: the care of the social body for the individual (creating the necessary relational conditions for healing), the integration of the individual through his or her encounter with the social body and its communal narratives (narrating the trauma), and the remaking of individuals through their participation in the social body and its practices (retemporalization). One additional aspect of the relation between individual and social bodies remains to be explored: the development of the individual as an agent of healing in the social body and in the world. As the insights of trauma scholars suggest, this represents another important component of retemporalization.

AGENTS OF NONVIOLENCE IN THE WORLD

As discussed in chapter 3, many trauma scholars observe that traumatized individuals often become agents of healing in the world by taking part in a "survivor mission," in which they participate in social action or intellectual pursuits designed to help others, such as political organizing or educating others about forms of harm such as sexual assault or domestic violence. These endeavors often function as an integral part of the healing process by giving survivors a sense of empowerment, a sense that they have made a contribution to the world that extends beyond their individual lives.

Many Christian theologians also underscore the importance of participating in social and political action, and some Christian communities provide rich resources for becoming involved in such efforts. As Amy Caiazza observes, people who take part in different forms of activism often first get involved in this work through their religious communities.[24] These communities provide a structure for social and political action, a group that shares a common interest in justice and, in some instances, a history of activism that provides valuable knowledge and experience. Moreover, religious communities offer motivation for pursuing this work; while their specific theological beliefs differ, they generally hold a basic sense of justice and human dignity that can inspire their members to join efforts that promote the well-being of all persons. Thus, for some traumatized persons, religious groups provide an important avenue for claiming a survivor mission and thereby acting as an agent of healing in the world.

Feminist theorist bell hooks indicates that people can become agents of change in the world, however, not only by participating in concrete movements for social transformation, but also simply by taking part in communities in which those who have been harmed by violence can survive and flourish. In *Talking Back: Thinking Feminist and Thinking Black*, she gives an account of healing from systemic violence that clarifies this point. Recognizing that systemic violence can become internalized in ways that are profoundly destructive to individuals and communities, hooks contends that healing from this violence involves resocialization, or remaking the socially constructed self. She explains that "Opposition is not enough. In that vacant space after one has resisted [the forces of oppression] there is still the necessity to become—to make oneself anew."[25]

For hooks, this process of making oneself anew takes place in communities that form on the margins of dominant society—not the marginality imposed upon people by oppressive structures but the marginality they choose as a site of resistance, of both "radical openness" and "radical possibility."[26] In these marginal spaces, communities can emerge in which people affirm one another and unlearn old ways of thinking and relating as they develop traditions and social practices that run counter to those of dominant society. Hooks argues that a central part of healing involves coming to understand how structures of domination function in one's life. This takes place as one remakes the self by developing an alternative worldview that maintains a critical stance in relation to normative social realities.[27] This alternative worldview, she adds, is fundamentally embodied. It involves not only words but also what one does, one's "habits of being."[28]

In hooks' view, the transformation of the individual self that can take place in such communities poses a challenge to broader social and political realities. If the self is (at least partly) socially constructed and therefore always engaged in larger social structures, then its remaking challenges these structures by resisting the conditions of domination they sanction and support.[29] The self, therefore, is itself a locus for political struggle or revolution; its healing from violence and oppression—its reclaiming of wholeness—constitutes an act of political resistance and transformation.[30] Thus, the healing of the self, the formation of community, and the transformation of social and political structures are not three different realities that take place in a temporally linear or sequential fashion. They are instead three dimensions of the same reality.

Translated into theological terms, hooks' analysis suggests that for the church to transform violence that is internal to its members, it must live as a community that participates in their social formation, constructing them differently than dominant culture. In many ways, this vision of Christian community resonates with Yoder's understanding of the church as an alternative community defined by the commitment its members have made with each other and with God. As such a community, the church is engaged in the reconstitution of identities, as its members collectively create a counter-cultural consciousness and ways of living that challenge the dominant structures of society. Like hooks, Yoder acknowledges the connection between the creation of such communities and the transformation of the world. He sees the construction of an alternative community as itself an act of political opposition to the powers, an act in which the church resists the powers by refusing to allow itself to be colonized by them. While Yoder does not discuss the healing of the self and its connection to the formation of community and transformation of broader social and political realities, his theological framework fits nicely with hooks' theoretical one.

Both Yoder and hooks, then, broaden the terms of what it means to act as an agent of change in the world. They suggest that being an agent of transformation is not simply a matter of what one does but also the kind of person one is. Put differently, becoming a person not colonized by the powers and principalities is itself an act of resistance. For some trauma survivors, it may bring additional hope to recognize that political action and the healing of the self are not dichotomous realities. Specifically, this recognition may enable them to realize that when they act as agents of their own healing by participating in the church's communal construction of a new eschatological identity, they contribute to the transformation of the world, albeit in small ways that often remain difficult to identify. By participating in the church's life and worship, survivors enact a different kind of survivor mission, one that challenges the violence of the powers by resisting its ongoing effects. This, in turn, makes a contribution to the world that extends beyond the change they experience in their individual lives.

While the healing of the self constitutes an act of political resistance in its own right, many survivors also benefit from participating in concrete movements for social change. As Herman observes, some traumatized persons find that such action provides a way they can continue to develop their "new" selves, establish additional life-giving relationships, and rebuild their sense of self-worth.[31] Identifying the interconnections between the healing of the self, the formation of community, and the transformation of the world thus does not imply that activism or other survivor missions are unimportant. Rather, it simply indicates that by participating in the alternative community of the church—a community that exists both "for" and "against" the world—survivors already are part of a social body that contributes to the transformation of the world.

NONVIOLENCE REDEFINED

Throughout this book I have argued that the healing or transformation of internalized, traumatic violence represents an often-overlooked dimension of Christian nonviolence. In the historic peace churches, for example, discussions of nonviolence have typically focused on how Christians can resist and transform external violence by embodying pacifism and refusing to sanction state violence. In conversation with trauma studies, I have suggested that extending the definition of violence beyond external violence to include internal violence requires rethinking the meaning and practice of nonviolence. Specifically, I have proposed that Christian nonviolence includes as well the creation of a community in which traumatized persons can heal from traumatic violence through the narrative construction and collective enactment of an eschatological identity, and through participation in the revealed but not yet fully realized new aeon.

This reconceptualization of Christian nonviolence, however, remains incomplete without adding one additional component: the integration of nonviolence into the being of the church and those who constitute it. To describe nonviolence simply as the rejection or transformation of (external and internal) violence implies that nonviolence leads to the absence of violence. The insights of feminist theory encourage us to expand this view of nonviolence a step further. Many feminists criticize Western patterns of thinking that view the world through the lens of either-or dichotomies such as man vs. woman, good vs. evil, violence vs. nonviolence. They argue that these patterns of thinking privilege the first term over the second, turning the second into a mere reflection of the first and robbing it of any independent meaning. From this perspective, understanding violence and nonviolence as dichotomous allows nonviolence no identity of its own. Feminist theory thus would encourage us to see nonviolence as not just a lack of violence but rather as something that has its own positive content. In the context of structural violence, nonviolence involves not only altering violent structures so that they no longer perpetrate violence, but also creating new structures that foster peace and reconciliation. In the context of violence that is internal to socially constructed people and communities, it entails not only transforming this violence, but also integrating nonviolence into their being.

Yoder's view of Christian community points to a way that nonviolence can become part of the being of the church and its members. Recall that for Yoder, the church is an alternative community that participates in the social formation of its members. Christians are shaped partly by the story of Jesus' nonviolent resistance to the powers as they reenact or perform this story through their life and worship. This vision of the church opens up the possibility that people can be constructed in a way that not only transforms internalized violence but also integrates nonviolence into their identity and being. As Christians shape their lives around this story that they hear and tell, the nonviolence of Jesus becomes part of the spirit of the church and of the people who constitute it. This integration of nonviolence into the church, however, is not a process the church completes on its own. Recall again Yoder's claim that God is also active in the church's communal performance of its practices.[32]

While Yoder's work offers resources for understanding how Christians might transform internalized violence and integrate nonviolence, he never explicitly discusses this matter. These issues find more concrete expression in the writings of another theologian of nonviolence, Martin Luther King, Jr. In "The Current Crisis in Race Relations," King identifies hatred as a form of internal violence that can become embedded in those who experience racism on an ongoing basis. He recognizes the destructive potential of this internalized violence, its capacity to destroy not only one's soul but also one's ability to work toward authentic social transformation. Thus, King argues, "Along the way of life, someone must have enough sense and morality to cut off the chain of hate by projecting the ethics of love into the center of our lives."[33]

Though the internal violence King refers to differs in some ways from the internal violence that trauma theorists describe, his brief discussion makes a crucial point: The communal practice of nonviolence involves forming people in such a way that nonviolence becomes integral to who they are. Nonviolence, put simply, becomes the space out of which they think and act. A pledge that King used for his followers in the 1963 sit-in demonstrations in Birmingham implicitly makes this point. Designed to prepare the demonstrators to seek change without using physical force, it outlines ten commandments that the demonstrators were to follow.[34] Heading the list are the commands to "meditate daily on the teachings and life of Jesus" and "remember always that the nonviolent movement in Birmingham seeks justice and reconciliation—not victory."[35] Surprisingly, refraining from violence does not show up on the list until number eight. King's choice to use a set of commandments structured in this way suggests that to refrain from violence, one's character must be formed in a particular way. More specifically, it suggests that to stop cycles of violence we must find ways for people to transform internalized violence and to integrate nonviolence into their identities.

For King, the biblical narratives contain rich resources for accomplishing this goal. These narratives provide the foundation for his theological vision of God and humanity as well as for the concrete enactment of that vision in the civil rights movement. King deeply believes that God created all human beings to be with each other and not separate from each other. He envisions us as one humanity, intended to live together as a diverse, integrated community marked by personal and social relationships of love, justice, and hope. In his view, the story of Jesus' crucifixion provides the catalyst for this idea. King understands the cross as both "an eternal expression of the lengths to which God goes to restore broken human community" and as a model for how Christians should live their own lives: committed to the rule of love and confident in God's power to provide the resources they need to face the challenges of life.[36]

King's analysis indicates that the internalization of nonviolence does not replace nonviolent direct action but serves as a foundation for it. For the Christian community (and for other communities) to sustain participation in social justice efforts, its members must have a sense of agency and wholeness as well as a vision of hope that inspires them to persist even in the face of perceived defeat. The church, then, can function as a powerful advocate for change in the world only if it works to internalize nonviolence and thereby create agents empowered to engage in the struggle—agents who not only experience the healing of their own injuries but also embody empathy, compassion, and a vision of the future that is different from the present.

SITES OF VIOLENCE, SITES OF GRACE

The formation of a community that creates nonviolent persons represents an integral part of what it means for the church "to be the church." If, as Yoder observes, nonviolence constitutes the cornerstone of the Christian faith, then we cannot ignore this crucial aspect of the church's life and mission. At the same time, we must recognize that this does not represent all of what it means for the church to be the church. To understand the Christian community as simply a community of "wounded healers" ignores both the multiple tasks of its ministry and the many ways it perpetrates violence.[37] The transformation of internal violence and the integration of nonviolence represent just part of the church's identity and mission, a part it does not always faithfully embody.

When the church does live into this calling, though, it reveals one way in which Christian communities and their individual members can be not only sites of violence but also sites of grace. Simply by living into the life to which they are called, these communities that manifest and offer God's grace to trauma survivors and their witnesses. By constructing voluntary and egalitarian relationships in which people hear each others' stories, by performing the narratives of Jesus through communal practices, and by embodying an alternative vision of the future, Christian communities manifest God's grace and enact an integral component of Christian nonviolence.

As a site of grace, the church is enabled to live out the particular story that shapes its life, the story of the one who breaks the link between the self as site of violence and the self as agent of violence. In breaking this link, Jesus ushered in a new beginning, a new age in which the powers no longer enjoy unchallengeable reign, although they do continue to have destructive effects in the world. Refusing to be made over into the violent image of the powers, he lives as the first fruits of a restored humanity, as the one who opens up the possibility of new life for us. Through its communal performance of his story, the church participates in this life he makes possible and thereby embodies a new eschatological identity: an identity that manifests the grace of his nonviolent spirit.

This suggestion that the church can be formed as a site of grace does not imply that the community's enactment of a nonviolent identity makes the violence within the church and its members simply disappear. If violence and nonviolence do not exist in dichotomous relation, then they can coexist within selves and communities; the presence of one does not cancel out the other. God's redemptive grace, as manifest in and through human communities, can transform the violence that is internal to selves and communities, but this transformation is an ongoing process.

All human beings can embody both violence and nonviolence. The traumatic violence that I have explored gives us one particularly acute example of how people can internalize violence, but human beings need not be traumatized to be constructed as sites of violence. In North America we watch violent movies, consume media images that are racist, sexist, and classist, and see daily news reports of war-torn regions. We do not remain unaffected by this violence. Rather, it becomes integral to our identities, informing how we think, act, and see the world. To put it in language that the Christian traditions have used, human beings are profoundly broken, even as they are regenerated by God's grace. The transformation and redemption that grace effects awaits a future consummation.[38] In this life we are both fragmented and whole, broken and redeemed.

The church, then, does not completely disentangle itself from the violence of the world. In Yoder's terms, the "alternative" character of the church does not mean that it simply sits over-against the world. Rather, the relation between church and world is much more complex. The brokenness of the world manifests itself in the church, even as the church strives to embody an alternative to the world's violence and oppression. Given the interrelatedness of church and world, one can argue, as Yoder does, that Christians need an ongoing critical process in which the church reflects on its own identity, asking how it might live more faithfully in the midst of its brokenness.[39]

In the context of violence that has become internal to the church and its members, this reflection entails considering the ways in which the church concretely practices its faith. In attending to the structures of its ordinary liturgical and social life, making changes where necessary, the church can transform internalized violence and integrate nonviolence into its being. This attention to its social life is crucial because, as Yoder points out, nonviolence is not merely something the church verbally proclaims but also something it does, an embodied way of life for the whole community. Note that in exploring how the church can embody this life through the normal course of its activities and worship, I do not mean to imply that it is easy or requires no special commitment. The decision to participate in a community that lives out the story of Jesus is not one to make lightly since, as Yoder observes, this life can prove costly indeed.

In addition to exploring how the church addresses trauma through its "normal" life and worship, one could consider "extraordinary" measures Christian communities might take to deal with trauma's impact on the lives of its members. For example, some have analyzed the ways in which religious rituals designed specifically to address traumatic injuries can help persons to heal.[40] Others argue that the church can assist survivors of violence by organizing education forums that raise consciousness about violence and address strategies for resisting and preventing it.[41] While such measures may prove helpful for some persons, they were not the focus of this book.

Additional work that explores ways in which Christian communities can address internal violence, especially that which stems from trauma, is much needed. For many years the church has struggled with trauma, and like other human communities it will continue to do so for many more. The theological reflections offered here do not provide a resolution to the "problem" of trauma or simple answers for how the church can help people recover, for there are no such answers. The Christian community merely stands as one among many in the world, each of which has its own potential resources.

While the church's resources do not assist all traumatized persons who seek help, they do prove beneficial for some. The insights of trauma studies, I have argued, give us a language and conceptuality for understanding how. My hope is that the reflections in this book will assist Christian communities currently struggling with trauma, and perhaps even give those not presently thinking about it a framework for considering how their communal life and worship contributes (or fails to contribute) to the creation of a context in which traumatized persons can survive and flourish.

While the church will never fully disentangle itself from violence, it can engage in an ongoing process of transforming internalized violence and integrating nonviolence into the community and those who constitute it. Through its life and worship, the church can live as an alternative community that participates in the social construction of its members, such that they become persons and communities who are not only sites of violence but also sites of grace. In so doing, it enacts a new eschatological identity that manifests signs of both violence and nonviolence: the identity of the risen Christ who bears the wounds of crucifixion.

NOTES

1. Jane Miller [pseudo.], conversation with the author, New Haven, CT, July 7, 2003.

2. Note two other important differences between the eschatological retemporalization that I am describing and the overlapping of times that trauma scholars discuss: First, in eschatological retemporalization the community, rather than merely the individual, is the site of this overlapping. Second, the voluntary character of Christian community suggests that in the church, people choose to participate in this overlapping of aeons. This affirms rather than undermines their agency.

3. See Herman, *Trauma and Recovery*, 202.

4. Jane Miller [pseudo.], conversation with the author, July 7, 2003.

5. Jane Miller [pseudo.], conversation with the author, July 7, 2003.

6. My reflections on memory, imagination, Christian eschatology, and the traumatized self are informed by Jill Carlson Colwell's presentation, "'Anticipatory Memory': Christian Eschatology and the Traumatized Self," presented to the Yale Doctoral Theology Seminar, December 12, 2001.

7. Kirmayer, "Landscapes of Memory," 174.

8. Procter-Smith, *In Her Own Rite*, 36.

9. Kirmayer, "Landscapes of Memory," 176.

10. Trevor Hart, "Imagination for the Kingdom of God?" in *God Will Be All in All: The Eschatology of Jürgen Moltmann*, ed. Richard Bauckham (Edinburgh, Scotland: T & T Clark, 1999), 54–55.

11. Hart, "Imagination for the Kingdom of God?" 55.

12. On the memory of the future, see Johann Baptist Metz, *Faith in History and Society: Toward a Practical Fundamental Theology*, translated by David Smith (New York: The Seabury Press, 1980), 100–118.

13. Yoder, *Body Politics*, 72–73.

14. Hart,"Imagination for the Kingdom of God," 75.

15. Colwell, "'Anticipatory Memory': Christian Eschatology and the Traumatized Self."

16. Colwell, "'Anticipatory Memory': Christian Eschatology and the Traumatized Self."

17. Hart, "Imagination for the Kingdom of God," 68.

18. This account of the relation between the new aeon and the old emphasizes the discontinuity between the two. Yet, it is important also to stress their continuity. As I have been arguing, for the memory of God's future to function as a resource for hope and healing, trauma survivors need to see this future as theirs. From a theological perspective, one can underscore this continuity by claiming that the new aeon does not replace or destroy the old but rather renews it through God's Spirit, even as it brings something that transcends any capacities within the old. The relation between these two aeons is thus one of both continuity and discontinuity. See Hart, "Imagination for the Kingdom of God," 65–68, and Jürgen Moltmann, *Theology of Hope* (New York: Harper & Row, 1967).

19. Yoder, *The Original Revolution*, 58–62.

20. Shannon Craigo-Snell, "Command Performance," 479.

21. Stephanie Paulsell, "Honoring the Body," in *Practicting Our Faith: A Way of Life for a Searching People,*" ed. Dorothy C. Bass (San Francisco: Jossey-Bass Publishers, 1997), 16.

22. These practices, of course, take place within the context of a tradition that has had an ambivalent relationship to the body. As Paulsell observes, some Christians have held a positive view of the body, claiming it as a locus for divine activity. Others have seen the body as "scandalous and repugnant" ("Honoring the Body," 16–18). For trauma survivors who have had their bodies violated, the latter view can prove particularly damaging insofar as it may reinforce their own negative views of their bodies.

23. Paulsell, "Honoring the Body," 16.

24. Patricia Hill Collins, "The Ties That Bind: Women's Public Vision for Politics, Religion, and Civil Society" (Washington, DC: Institute for Women's Policy Research, 2005), 3.

25. Bell Hooks, "The Politics of Radical Black Subjectivity," *Yearning: Race, Gender, and Cultural Politics* (Boston: South End Press, 1990),15.

26. Hooks, "Choosing the Margin as a Space of Radical Openness," in *Yearning*, 149.

27. Hooks, "Choosing the Margin as a Space of Radical Openness," 150.

28. Hooks, "Choosing the Margin as a Space of Radical Openness," 149.

29. Hooks also notes that selves that are whole can more effectively sustain engagement in active political struggle. See *Sisters of the Yam: Black Women and Self-Recovery* (Boston: South End Press, 1993), 14–15.

30. As do some trauma theorists, hooks acknowledges that the language of "self-recovery" is problematic because it implies that there exists a whole or coherent self that survivors can recover. Some question whether this is true for those who have experienced exploitation or dehumanization since a very young age. Hooks addresses this objection by arguing that the "self" is not an individual "I" but "the coming together of many 'I's.'" The self embodies "collective reality past and present, family and community"—voices that are silenced under conditions of domination. Those who have experienced a lifetime of oppression, then, can recover their wholeness by coming to know their history, so that their "field of vision is no longer shaped and determined solely by the condition of domination." See Hooks, *Talking Back*, 30–31.

31. Herman, *Trauma and Recovery*, 207–211.

32. Yoder, *Body Politics*, 72–73.

33. King, *A Testament of Hope*, 85–86.

34. *The Words of Martin Luther King, Jr.* Selected by Coretta Scott King (New York: New Market Press, 1983), 74.

35. *The Words of Martin Luther King, Jr.*, 74.

36. See King, "A Walk through the Holy Land," sermon given March 29, 1959, at Dexter Baptist Church in Montogomery, AL, and King, "Revolution and Redemption," address given April 16, 1964, to the European Baptist Assembly, Amsterdam, Holland. Both texts are in Martin Luther King, Jr., Papers, Martin Luther King, Jr., Center for Nonviolent Social Change, Atlanta, GA.

37. See Henri Nouwen, *The Wounded Healer* (New York: Doubleday Publishing, 1979).

38. Christians believe that even in the eschatological future, this brokenness will be transformed but not erased. Recall the image of the resurrected Christ who still bears the wounds of crucifixion.

39. Yoder, "The Believers Church and the Arms Race," in *For the Nations*, 157.

40. See Rebecca, Lea Nicoll Kramer, and Susan A. Lukey, "Spirit Song: The Use of Christian Healing Rites in Trauma Recovery," *Treating Abuse Today* 5, no. 6 (November/December 1995): 39–47. See also Rosemary Radford Ruther, *Women- Church* (San Francisco: Harper & Row, 1985), 149–81.

41. For example, see Traci C. West, *Wounds of the Spirit: Black Women, Violence, and Resistance Ethics* (New York: New York University Press, 1999), 195–96.

Bibliography

Abramson, A. and G. Lucido. "Childhood Sexual Experience and Bulimia." *Addictive Behaviors* 16 (1991): 529–32.

Adler, Lisa and L.H.M. Ling. "From Practice to Theory: Towards a Dissident-Feminist Reconstruction of Nonviolence." *Gandhi Marg: Journal of the Gandhi Peace Foundation*, 16, no. 4 (January–March 1995): 462–80.

Alexander, Debra Whiting. *Children Changed by Trauma: A Healing Guide*. Oakland, CA: New Harbinger Publications, Inc., 1999.

Allen, Jon G. *Coping with Trauma: A Guide to Self-Understanding*. Washington, DC: American Psychiatric Publishing, Inc., 1995.

American Psychiatric Association. *Diagnostic and Statistical Manual of Mental Disorders: DSM-IV*. 4th ed. Washington, DC: American Psychiatric Association, 1994.

Apsey, Lawrence S. "How Transforming Power Has Been Used in the Past by Early Christians," in *Nonviolence in Theory and Practice*. Ed. by Robert L. Holmes, 27–28. Prospect Heights, IL: Waveland Press, 1990.

Bainton, Roland H. *Christian Attitudes Toward War and Peace: A Historical Survey and Critical Re-evaluation*. Nashville, TN: Abingdon Press, 1960.

Barstown, Anne Llewellyn. "Nonviolent Interventions: A Response to Terrorism." *Church and Society* 94, no. 5 (May–June 2004): 25–33.

Beasley-Murry, Paul. *Power for God's Sake: Power and Abuse in the Local Church*. Carlisle: Paternoster, 1998.

Berkhof, Hendrikus. *Christ and the Powers*. Trans. John Howard Yoder. Scottdale, PA: Herald Press, 1977.

Bernt, Hagen. *Non-violence in the World Religions: Vision and Reality*. Trans. by John Bowden. London: SCM Press, 1998.

Beste, Jennifer. *God and the Victim: Traumatic Intrusions on Grace and Freedom*. New York: Oxford University Press, 2007.

Bloom, Sandra. *Creating Sanctuary: Toward an Evolution of Sane Societies*. New York: Routledge, 1997.

Bloom, Sandra L. and Michael Reichert. *Bearing Witness: Violence and Collective Responsibility.* New York: The Haworth Maltreatment and Trauma Press, 1998.
Brison, Susan. *Aftermath: Violence and the Remaking of a Self.* Princeton, NJ: Princeton University Press, 2002.
Brock, Rita Nakashima. *Journeys by Heart: A Christology of Erotic Power.* New York: Crossroad Publishing Company, 1988.
Brock, Rita Nakashima and Rebecca Ann Parker. *Proverbs of Ashes: Violence, Redemptive Suffering, and the Search for What Saves Us.* Boston: Beacon Press, 2001.
Brown Douglas, Kelly. *The Black Christ.* Maryknoll, NY: Orbis Books, 1993.
Brown, Joanne Carlson and Rebecca Parker. "For God So Loved the World?" in *Christianity, Patriarchy, and Abuse: A Feminist Critique.* Eds. Joanne Carlson Brown and Carole R. Bohn, 1–30. New York: Pilgrim Press, 1989.
Brown, Laura S. "Not Outside the Range: One Feminist Perspective on Psychic Trauma," in *Trauma: Explorations in Memory.* Ed. Cathy Caruth, 100–112. Baltimore: The Johns Hopkins University Press, 1995.
Butler, Judith. "Contingent Foundations," in *Feminist Contentions: A Philosophical Exchange.* Ed. Seyla Benhabib et al. New York: Routledge, 1995.
——. *Gender Trouble: Feminism and the Subversion of Identity.* New York: Routledge, 1990.
Caiazza, Amy. *The Ties That Bind: Women's Public Vision for Politics, Religion, and Civil Society.* Washington, DC: Institute for Women's Policy Research, 2005.
Cameron, Catherine. *Resolving Childhood Trauma: A Long-Term Study of Abuse Survivors.* Thousand Oaks, CA: Sage Publications, 2000.
Carino, Kathi. "A Dark Room in My Mind." *Perspectives* 7 (September 1992): 9–12.
Carlson, Eve B., et al. "Relationships Between Traumatic Experiences and Symptoms of Posttraumatic Stress, Dissociation, and Amnesia," in *Trauma, Memory, and Dissociation.* Eds. J. Douglas Bremner and Charles R. Marmar, 205–27. Washington, DC: American Psychiatric Press, Inc., 1998.
Carter, Craig. *The Politics of the Cross: The Theology and Social Ethics of John Howard Yoder.* Grand Rapids, MI: Brazos Press, 2001.
Cohen, Tamar. "Motherhood Among Incest Survivors." *Child Abuse and Neglect* 19, no. 12 (2000): 1423–29.
Collins, Patricia Hill. "The Ties That Bind: Race, Gender and US Violence." *Ethnic and Racial Studies,* 21, issue 5 (Sept. 1998): 917–38.
Cooper-White, Pamela. *The Cry of Tamar: Violence Against Women and the Church's Response.* Minneapolis: Augsburg Fortress Press, 1995.
Cortright, David. *Gandhi and Beyond: Nonviolence for an Age of Terrorism.* Boulder, CO: Paradigm Publishers, 2006.
Craigo-Snell, Shannon. "Command Performance: Rethinking Performance Interpretation in the Context of Divine Discourse." *Modern Theology* 16 no. 4 (October 2000): 475–94.
Crysdale, Cynthia. *Embracing Travail: Retrieving the Cross Today.* New York: Continuum, 1999.
Culliton, Joseph, ed. *Non-violence—Central to Christian Spirituality: Perspectives from Scripture to the Present.* New York: The Edwin Mellon Press, 1982.
Deboe, James. "Personality-Splitting Trauma." *Perspectives* 7 (September 1992): 13–15.

Diagnostic and Statistical Manual of Mental Disorders: DSM-IV, Washington, DC: American Psychiatric Association, 1994.

Doehring, Carrie. *Internal Desecration: Traumatization and Representations of God.* Lanham, MD: University Press of America, 1993.

Douglass, James W. *The Nonviolent Coming of God.* Maryknoll, NY: Orbis Books, 1991.

Durnbaugh, Donald. *The Believers Church: The History and Character of Radical Reformation Protestantism.* New York: Macmillan, 1968.

Egendorf, Arthur. *Healing from War: Trauma and Transformation at Vietnam.* Boston: Houghton Mifflin, 1985.

Erikson, Kai. *A New Species of Trouble: Explorations in Disaster, Trauma, and Community.* New York: W. W. Norton & Company, 1994.

———. "Notes on Trauma and Community," in *Trauma: Explorations in Memory.* Ed. Cathy Caruth, 183–99. Baltimore, MD: The Johns Hopkins University Press, 1995.

Farwell, Nancy and Jamie B. Cole. "Community as a Context of Healing: Psychosocial Recovery of Children Affected by War and Political Violence." *International Journal of Mental Health,* 30, no. 4 (Winter 2001–2002): 19–41.

Felman, Shoshana and Dori Laub, M.D. *Testimony: Crises of Witnessing in Literature, Psychoanalysis, and History.* New York: Routledge, 1992.

Flax, Jane. *Thinking Fragments: Psychoanalysis, Feminism, and Postmodernism in the Contemporary West.* Berkeley, CA: The University of California Press, 1990.

Fortune, Marie M. "Forgiveness: The Last Step," in *Violence against Women and Children: A Christian Theological Sourcebook.* Eds. Carol J. Adams and Marie M. Fortune, 201–6. New York: Continuum, 1995.

———. *Is Nothing Sacred? When Sex Invades the Pastoral Relationship.* San Francisco, CA: Harper & Row, 1989.

Fortune, Marie M. and James N. Poling. *Sexual Abuse by Clergy: A Crisis for the Church.* Decatur, GA: Journal of Pastoral Care Publications, 1994.

Fuss, Diana. *Essentially Speaking: Feminism, Nature, and Difference.* New York: Routledge, 1989.

Gilfus, Mary E. "The Price of a Ticket: A Survivor-Centered Appraisal of Trauma Theory." *Violence Against Women,* 5, issue 11 (November 1999): 1238–57.

Gilmore, Leigh. *The Limits of Autobiography: Trauma and Testimony.* Ithaca, NY: Cornell University Press, 2000.

Goertz, Karein. "Transgenerational Representations of the Holocaust: From Memory to 'Post-Memory.'" *World Literature Today* 72 no. 1 (Winter 1998): 33–38.

Graham, Stephen A. "What Would Jesus Do About Terrorism? Christian Realism and Christian Pacifism." *Encounter* 65, no. 4 (Autumn 2004): 345–71.

Grant, Jacquelyn. *White Women's Christ and Black Women's Jesus: Feminist Christology and Womanist Response.* Atlanta: Scholars Press, 1989.

Gudorf, Christine. *Victimization: Examining Christian Complacency.* Philadelphia: Trinity Press International, 1992.

Gutierrez, Gustavo. *A Theology of Liberation: History, Politics, and Salvation.* Trans. and eds. Sister Caridad Inda and John Eagleson. Maryknoll, NY: Orbis Books, 1973. Reprinted 1988.

Haen, Craig and Kenneth H. Brannon. "Superheroes, Monsters, and Babies: Roles of Strength, Destruction, and Vulnerability for Emotionally Disturbed Boys." *The Arts in Psychotherapy* 29 (2002): 31–40.

Hagood, Maralynn M. *The Use of Art in Counseling Child and Adult Survivors of Sexual Abuse.* London: Jessica Kingsley Publishers, 2000.

Hakken, Janice. "The Good, the Bad, and the Ugly: Psychoanalytic and Cultural Perspectives on Forgiveness," in *Before Forgiving: Cautionary Views of Forgiveness in Psychotherapy*. Eds. Sharon Lamb and Jeffrie G. Murphy, 172–91. Oxford: Oxford University Press, 2002.

Hall, Terese A. "Spiritual Effects of Childhood Sexual Abuse in Adult Christian Women." *Journal of Psychology and Theology* 23, no. 2 (Summer 1995): 129–34.

Hart, Trevor. "Imagination for the Kingdom of God?" in *God Will Be All in All: The Eschatology of Jürgen Moltmann*. Ed. Richard Bauckham, 49–76. Edinburgh, Scotland: T & T Clark, 1999.

Harter, Susan. *The Construction of the Self: A Developmental Perspective.* New York: The Guilford Press, 1999.

Hartman, Saidiya. *Scenes of Subjection: Terror, Slavery, and Self-Making in Nineteenth-Century America.* New York: Oxford University Press, 1997.

Hastings, Tom H. *Nonviolent Response to Terrorism*. Jefferson, NC: McFarland & Company, 2004.

Hauerwas, Stanley. *The Peaceable Kingdom.* Notre Dame: The University of Notre Dame Press, 1983.

Heggen, Carolyn Holderread. *Sexual Abuse in Christian Homes and Churches.* Scottdale, PA: Herald Press, 1993.

Herman, Judith Lewis. "Complex PTSD: A Syndrome in Survivors of Prolonged and Repeated Trauma," in *Psychotraumatology: Key Papers and Core Concepts in Post-traumatic Stress.* Eds. George S. Everly, Jr. and Jeffrey M. Lating, 87–100. New York: Plenum Press, 1995.

———. *Trauma and Recovery.* New York: BasicBooks, 1992.

Heyward, Carter. "Nonviolent Ways." *Christianity and Crisis*, 53 (April 12, 1993): 81–82.

Hirsch, Herbert. *Genocide and the Politics of Memory: Studying Death to Preserve Life.* Chapel Hill, NC: University of North Carolina Press, 1995.

Holmes, Robert L. *Nonviolence in Theory and Practice.* Prospect Heights, IL: Waveland Press, Inc., 1990.

hooks, bell. *Sisters of the Yam: Black Women and Self-Recovery*. Boston: South End Press, 1993.

———. *Talking Back: Thinking Feminist, Thinking Black*. Boston: South End Press, 1989.

———. *Yearning: Race, Gender, and Cultural Politics*. Boston: South End Press, 1990.

Hopkins, Nancy Myer and Mark Laaser. *Restoring the Soul of a Church: Healing Congregations Wounded by Clergy Sexual Misconduct.* Washington, DC: Alban Institute, 1995.

Huebner, Chris K. "Mennonites and Narrative Theology: The Case of John Howard Yoder." *Conrad Grebel Review* 16 (Spring 1998): 15–38.

Hütter, Reinhold. "The Church: Midwife of History or Witness of the Eschaton?" *Journal of Religious Ethics* 18, no. 1 (Spring 1990): 27–54.

Janoff-Bulman, Ronnie. "Characterological Versus Behavioral Self-Blame: Inquiries into Depression and Rape," *Journal of Personality and Social Psychology* 37, no. 10 (1979): 1798–1809.

———. *Shattered Assumptions: Towards a New Psychology of Trauma*. New York: The Free Press, 1992.

Johnson, David Read. *Essays on the Creative Arts Therapies: Imaging the Birth of a Profession*. Springfield, IL: Charles C Thomas Publisher, 1999.

Jones L. Gregory. *Embodying Forgiveness: A Theological Analysis.* Grand Rapids, MI: Eerdmans, 1995.

Jones, Serene. "Emmaus Witnessing: Trauma and the Disordering of the Theological Imagination." *Union Seminary Quarterly Review* 55, no. 3–4 (2001): 113–28.

———. *Feminist Theory and Christian Theology: Cartographies of Grace.* Minneapolis: Fortress Press, 2000.

———. "Selving Faith: Feminist Theory and Feminist Theology Rethink the Self," in *Religion, Scholarship, and Higher Education*. Ed. Andrea Sterk, 142–49. Notre Dame, IN: The University of Notre Dame Press, 2002.

———. "Trauma and Grace." *Reflections*. Ed. Jamie L. Manson and published by Harold W. Attridge. New Haven, CT: Yale Divinity School (Winter 2004): 8–15.

Justice, William G. and Warren Lambert. "A Comparative Study of the Language People Use to Describe the Personalities of God and Their Earthly Parents." *The Journal of Pastoral Care,* 40, no. 2 (June 1986): 166–72.

Kane, Donna, Sharon E. Cheston, and Joanne Greer. "Perception of God by Survivors of Childhood Sexual Abuse: An Exploratory Study in an Underresearched Area." *Journal of Psychology and Theology* 21, no. 3 (1993): 228–37.

Keshgegian, Flora A. *Redeeming Memories: A Theology of Healing and Transformation.* Nashville, TN: Abingdon Press, 2000.

King, Martin Luther. "The Current Crisis in Race Relations," in *A Testament of Hope: The Essential Writings of Martin Luther King, Jr.* Ed. James Melvin Washington, 85–90. San Francisco: Harper & Row, 1986.

———. "The Drum Major Instinct," in *A Testament of Hope: The Essential Writings of Martin Luther King, Jr.* Ed. James Melvin Washington, 259–67. San Francisco: Harper & Row, 1986.

———. "Revolution and Redemption." Address given April 16, 1964, to the European Baptist Assembly. In Martin Luther King, Jr., Papers. Martin Luther King, Jr., Center for Nonviolent Social Change. Atlanta, GA.

"A Walk Through the Holy Land." Sermon given March 29, 1959, at Dexter Baptist Church. In the Martin Luther King, Jr. Papers. Martin Luther King, Jr., Center for Nonviolent Social Change. Atlanta, GA.

———. *Why We Can't Wait.* New York: Signet Classic, 2000 (first edition printed by Harper & Row, 1964).

The Words of Martin Luther King, Jr. Selected and introduced by Coretta Scott King. New York: New Market Press, 1984.

Kirk-Duggan, Cheryl A. *Exorcizing Evil: A Womanist Perspective on the Spirituals.* Maryknoll, NY: Orbis Books, 1997.

Kirmayer, Laurence. "Landscapes of Memory: Trauma, Narrative, and Dissociation," in *Tense Past: Cultural Essays in Trauma and Memory.* Eds. Paul Antze and Michael Lambek, 173–98. New York: Routledge, 1996.

Kleber, Rolf J., Charles R. Figley, and Berthold P. R. Gersons, eds. *Beyond Trauma: Cultural and Societal Dynamics.* New York: Plenum Press, 1995.

LaCapra, Domonick. *History and Memory after Auschwitz.* Ithaca, NY: Cornell University Press, 1998.

Lacugna, Catherine Mowry. *Freeing Theology: The Essentials of Theology in Feminist Perspective.* New York: HarperCollins, 1993.

Lamb, Sharon. "Reasons to Be Cautious about the Use of Forgiveness Psychotherapy," in *Before Forgiving: Cautionary Views of Forgiveness in Psychotherapy.* Eds. Sharon Lamb and Jeffrie G. Murphy, 3–16. Oxford: Oxford University Press, 2002.

———. *The Trouble with Blame: Victims, Perpetrators, and Responsibility.* Cambridge, MA: Harvard University Press, 1995.

———. "Women Abuse, and Forgiveness: A Special Case," in *Before Forgiving: Cautionary Views of Forgiveness in Psychotherapy.* Eds. Sharon Lamb and Jeffrie G. Murphy, 155–71. Oxford: Oxford University Press, 2002.

Langer, Lawrence. *Holocaust Testimonies: The Ruins of Memory.* New Haven, CT: Yale University Press, 1991.

Laub, Dori and Shoshana Fleman. *Testimony: Crises of Witnessing in Literature, Psychoanalysis, and History.* Eds. Shoshana Felman and Dori Laub, 57–74 and 75–92. New York: Routledge, 1992.

Lefkovitz, Lori Hope. "The Inherited Holocaust Memory and the Ethics of Ventriloquism." *The Kenyon Review* Ns 19 (Winter 1997): 34–43.

Lemoncelli, John and Andrew Carey. "The Psychospiritual Dynamics of Adult Survivors of Abuse." *Counseling and Values* 40 (1996): 175–84.

Leslie, Kristen J. *When Violence Is No Stranger: Pastoral Counseling with Survivors of Acquaintance Rape.* Minneapolis: Fortress Press, 2003.

Levi, Primo. *Survival in Auschwitz.* Trans. Stuart Woolf. New York: Collier Books, Macmillan Publishing Company, 1961.

Leys, Ruth. *Trauma: A Genealogy.* Chicago: The University of Chicago Press, 2000.

Lifton, Robert J. *The Protean Self: Human Resilience in an Age of Fragmentation.* New York: Basicbooks, 1993.

Manlowe, Jennifer. *Faith Born of Seduction: Sexual Trauma, Body Image, and Religion.* New York: New York University Press, 1995.

McAllister, Pam, ed. *Reweaving the Web of Life: Feminism and Nonviolence.* Philadelphia: New Society Publishers, 1982.

McClendon, James W. Jr. "The Voluntary Church in the Twenty-First Century," in *The Believers Church: A Voluntary Church.* Ed. William H. Brackney, 179–98. Kitchener, Ontario: Pandora Press, 1998.

Means, Jeffrey and Mary Ann Nelson. *Trauma and Evil: Healing the Wounded Soul.* Minneapolis: Augsburg Fortress, 2000.

Meekums, Bonnie. *Creative Group Therapy for Women Survivors of Child Sexual Abuse.* London: Jessica Kingsley Publishers, 2000.

Mercadante, Linda. "Anguish: Unraveling Sin And Victimization." *Anglican Theological Review* 82:2 (Spring 2000): 283–302.

———. "A Spirituality 'After.'" *Newsletter of the Interfaith Sexual Trauma Institute* 5:1 (January 1999): 3–5.

Metz, Johannes Baptist. *Faith in History and Society: Toward a Practical Fundamental Theology.* Translated by David Smith. New York: Seabury Press, 1980.

Miller, William Robert. *Nonviolence: A Christian Interpretation*. New York: Schocken Books, 1964.

Mills, Letty and Judith C. Daniluk. "Her Body Speaks: The Experience of Dance Therapy for Women Survivors of Child Sexual Abuse." *Journal of Counseling and Development* 80, no. 1 (Winter 2002): 77–85.

Minow, Martha. *Between Vengeance and Forgiveness*. Boston: Beacon Press, 1998.

Mishara, Aaron. "Narrative and Psychotherapy—the Phenomenology of Healing." *American Journal of Psychotherapy* 49 (Spring 1995): 180–95.

Moltmann, Jürgen. *The Coming of God: Christian Eschatology*. Trans. Margaret Kohl. Minneapolis: Fortress Press, 1996.

———. *The Crucified God: The Cross of Christ as the Foundation and Criticism of Christian Theology*. Trans. R.A. Wilson and John Bowden. Minneapolis: Fortress Press, 1993.

———. *Theology of Hope: On the Ground and the Implications of a Christian Eschatology*. New York: Harper & Row, 1967.

Moore, Allison Mauel. "Moral Agency of Women in a Battered Women's Shelter." *Violence Against Women*. Eds. Carol J. Adams and Marie M. Fortune, 172–84. New York: Continuum, 1995.

Morrison, Toni. *Beloved*. New York: Penguin Putnam, Inc., 1987.

———. *The Bluest Eye*. New York: Alfred A. Knopf, Inc., 1993.

Musto, Ronald G. *The Catholic Peace Tradition*. Maryknoll, NY: Orbis Books, 1986.

Nelson Dunfee, Susan. "The Sin of Hiding." *Soundings* 65 (Fall 1982): 316–27.

Nouwen, Henri. *The Wounded Healer*. Doubleday Publishing, 1979.

Nuttall, Geoffrey F. *Christian Pacifism in History*. Oxford: Blackwell, 1953.

Ortner, Sherry and Harriet Whitehead, eds. *Sexual Meanings, the Cultural Construction of Gender and Sexuality*. New York: Cambridge University Press, 1981.

Overcash, Wendy, et al. "Coping with Crises: An Examination of the Impact of Traumatic Events on Religious Beliefs." *The Journal of Genetic Psychology* 157 (December 1996): 455–64.

Painter, Nell. *Soul Murder and Slavery*. Waco: Baylor University Press, 1995.

Palmer, R. et al. "Childhood Sexual Experiences with Adults Reported by Women with Eating Disorders: An Extended Series." *British Journal of Psychiatry* 156 (1990): 669–703.

Papanikolaou, Aristotle. "Person, *Kenosis* and Abuse: Hans Urs von Balthasar and Feminist Theologies in Convesation." *Modern Theology* 19:1 (January 2003): 357–85.

Park, Andrew Sung and Susan L. Nelson, ed. *The Other Side of Sin: Woundedness from the Perspective of the Sinned-Against*. Albany: State University of New York Press, 2001.

Paulsell, Stephanie. "Honoring the Body," in *Practicing Our Faith: A Way of Life for a Searching People*. Ed. Dorothy C. Bass: 13–27. San Francisco: Jossey-Bass Publishers, 1997.

Pellauer, Mary D. and Susan Brooks Thistlethwaite. "Conversation on Grace and Healing: Perspectives from the Movement to End Violence Against Women," in *Lift Every Voice: Constructing Christian Theologies from the Underside*. Eds. Susan Brooks Thistlethwaite and Mary Potter Engel, 177–92. Maryknoll, NY: Orbis Books, 1998

Penner, Carol. "Content to Suffer: An Exploration of Mennonite Theology from the Context of Violence Against Women," in *Peace Theology and Violence Against Women*. Ed. Elizabeth G. Yoder, 99–111. Elkhart, IN: Institute of Mennonite Studies, 1992.

———. "Sexual Assault, Resurrection, and the Healing Community." *Consensus* 28, no. 2 (2002): 49–60.

Plank, Karl A. *Mother of the Wire Fence: Inside and Outside the Holocaust.* Louisville: Westminster John Knox Press, 1994.

Plaskow, Judith. *Sex, Sin, and Grace: Women's Experience and the Theologies of Reinhold Niebuhr and Paul Tillich.* Washington, DC: University Press of America, 1980.

Plumwood, Val. *Feminism and the Mastery of Nature.* London: Routledge, 1993.

Potter Engel, Mary. "Evil, Sin, and the Violation of the Vulnerable," in *Lift Every Voice: Constructing Christian Theologies from the Underside.* Eds. Susan Brooks Thistlethwaite and Mary Potter Engel, 159–71. Maryknoll, NY: Orbis Books, 1998.

Procter-Smith, Majorie. *in Her Own Rite: Constructing Feminist Liturgical Tradition.* Nashville: Abingdon Press, 1990.

Puka, Bill. "Forgoing Forgiveness," in *Before Forgiving: Cautionary Views of Forgiveness in Psychotherapy.* Eds. Sharon Lamb and Jeffrie G. Murphy, 136–52. Oxford: Oxford University Press, 2002.

Radford Ruether, Rosemary. "Feminism and Peace." *The Christian Century* 100:25 (August 31 and September 7, 1983): 771–76.

Rebecca, Lea Nicoll Kramer and Susan A. Lukey. "Spirit Song: The Use of Christian Healing Rites in Trauma Recovery." *Treating Abuse Today* 5 and 6 (November/December 1995 and January/February 1996): 39–47.

Redmond, Sheila. "God Died and Nobody Gave a Funeral." *Pastoral Psychology* 45, no. 1 (Spring 1996): 41–47.

Rizzuto, Ana Maria. *Birth of the Living God: A Psychoanalytic Study.* Chicago: The University of Chicago Press, 1979.

Roberts, Janine. "Beyond Words: The Power of Rituals," in *Beyond Talk Therapy: Using Movement and Expressive Techniques in Clinical Practice.* Ed. Daniel J. Wiener, 55–78. Washington, DC: American Psychological Association, 1999.

Root, Maria P.P. "Reconstructing the Impact of Trauma on Personality," in *Personality and Psychopathology: Feminist Reappraisals.* Eds. Laura S. Brown and Mary Ballou, 229–61. New York: The Guilford Press, 1992.

Rowell, James L. "Has Nonviolent Religion Been Trumped?" *Theology Today* 63 no. 2 (July 2006): 223–26.

Ruether, Rosemary Radford. *Women-Church: Theology and Practice of Feminist Liturgical Communities.* San Francisco: Harper & Row, 1985.

Russell, Diana. *The Secret Trauma: Incest in the Lives of Girls and Women.* New York: Basicbooks, 1986.

Russell, Diana E.H. and Rebecca Morris Bolen. *The Epidemic of Rape and Child Sexual Abuse in the United States.* Thousand Oaks, CA: Sage Publications, Inc., 2000.

Russell, Letty M., ed. *The Church with AIDS: Renewal in the Midst of Crisis.* Louisville: Westminster John Knox Press, 1990.

———. *The Church in the Round: Feminist Interpretation of the Church.* Louisville: Westminster John Knox Press, 1993.

———. *Household of Freedom.* Philadelphia: Westminster, 1987.

Russell, Letty M. and Shannon Clarkson, eds. *Dictionary of Feminist Theologies.* Louisville: Westminster John Knox Press, 1996.

Ryan, Gail. "Victim to Victimizer: Rethinking Victim Treatment." *Journal of Interpersonal Violence* 4, no. 3 (1989): 325–41.

Saiving, Valerie. "The Human Situation: A Feminine View," in *Womanspirit Rising: A Feminist Reader in Religion*. Eds. Carol P. Christ and Judith Plaskow. New York: Harper & Row, 1979.

Scarry, Elaine. *The Body in Pain: The Making and Unmaking of the World*. New York: Oxford University Press, 1985.

Schaefer, Charles E., ed. *The Therapeutic Powers of Play*. Northvale, NJ: Jason Aronson, Inc., 1993.

Schüssler Fiorenza, Elisabeth. *Discipleship of Equals: A Critical Feminist Ekklesialogy of Liberation*. New York: Crossroad, 1993.

Shengold, Leonard. *Soul Murder: The Effects of Childhood Abuse and Deprivation*. New York: Fawcett Columbine, 1989.

Shupe, Anson D., William A. Stacey, and Susan E. Darnell, eds. *Bad Pastors: Clergy Misconduct in Modern America*. New York: New York University Press, 2000.

Simonds, Susan L. *Bridging the Silence: Nonverbal Modalities in the Treatment of Adult Survivors of Childhood Sexual Abuse*. New York: W. W. Norton & Company, Inc., 1994.

Smith, Archie Jr. *The Relational Self: Ethics and Therapy from a Black Church Perspective*. Nashville, TN: Abingdon, 1982.

Squire, L. *Memory and the Brain*. New York: Oxford University Press, 1987.

Stapert, John. "God Enters Dark Closets." *Perspectives* 7 (September 1992): 16–18.

Stark, Evan. *Coercive Control*. New York: Oxford University Press, 2007.

Tal, Kalí. *Worlds of Hurt: Reading the Literatures of Trauma*. New York: Cambridge University Press, 1996.

Tellenbach, Gerd. *The Church in Western Europe from the Tenth to the Early Twelfth Century*. Cambridge, England: Cambridge University Press, 1993.

Terr, Lenore. "Childhood Traumas: An Outline and Overview." *American Journal of Psychiatry* 148 (1991): 10–20.

———. *Too Scared to Cry: Psychic Trauma in Childhood*. New York: Basicbooks, 1990.

Terrell, JoAnne Marie. *Power in the Blood? The Cross in African American Experience*. Maryknoll, NY: Orbis Books, 1998.

Toole, David. *Waiting for Godot in Sarajevo*. Boulder, CO: Westview Press, 1998.

Turner, Victor. *Dramas, Fields, and Metaphors: Symbolic Action in Human Society*. New York: Cornell University Press, 1974.

Urquiza, Anthony and Lisa Marie Keating. "The Prevalence of Sexual Victimization of Males," in *The Sexually Abused Male*. Ed. Mic Hunter, 1, 105–35. Lexington, MA: Lexington Books, 1990.

Van der Kolk, Bessel. *Psychological Trauma*. Washington, DC: American Psychiatric Press, 1987.

Van der Kolk, Bessel, Lars Weisaeth, and Onno van der Hart. *Traumatic Stress: The Effects of Overwhelming Experience on Mind, Body, and Society*. New York: The Guilford Press, 1996.

Vandervelde, George. "Believers Church Ecclesiology as Ecumenical Challenge," in *The Believers Church: A Voluntary Church*. Ed. by William H. Brackney, 199–216. Kitchener, Ontario: Pandora Press, 1998.

Vento, Johann M. "Violence, Trauma, and Resistance: A Feminist Appraisal of Metz's Mysticism of Suffering Unto God." *Horizons* 29: 1 (2002): 7–22.

Waites, Elizabeth A. *Trauma and Survival: Post-Traumatic and Dissociative Disorders in Women.* New York: W. W. Norton & Company, 1993.

Walker, Alice. *The Color Purple.* New York: Pocket Books, 1992.

Wallis, Jim. "Hard Questions for Peacemakers: Theologians of Nonviolence Wrestle with How to Resist Terrorism." *Sojourners Magazine* 31, no. 1 (January–February 2002): 29–33.

Weaver, J. Denny. "The Yoder Legacy: Whither the Second Generation?" *The Mennonite Quarterly Review* 77, no. 3 (July 2003): 451–71.

Weaver Fancisco, Patricia. *Telling: A Memoir of Rape and Recovery.* New York: Cliff Street Books, 1999.

West, Traci. *Wounds of the Spirit: Black Women, Violence, and Resistance Ethics.* New York: New York University Press, 1999.

Westerlund, Elaine. *Women's Sexuality after Childhood Incest.* New York: W.W. Norton, 1992.

Wiesel, Elie. *From the Kingdom of Memory.* New York: Schocken Books, 1990.

Williams, Delores. *Sisters in the Wilderness: The Challenge of Womanist God-Talk.* Maryknoll, NY: Orbis Books, 1993.

Williams, George Huntston. *The Radical Reformation.* Philadelphia: Westminster, 1962.

Wilson, Melba. *Crossing the Boundary: Black Women Survive Incest.* Seattle, WA: Seal Press, 1993.

Yoder, Carolyn. *The Little Book of Trauma Healing: When Violence Strikes and Community Security Is Threatened.* Intercourse, PA: Good Books, Inc., 2005.

Yoder, John Howard. *Body Politics: Five Practices of the Christian Community before the Watching World.* Nashville: Discipleship Resources, 1992, reprinted 1997.

———. *Christian Attitudes to War, Peace, and Revolution: A Companion to Bainton.* Elkhart, IN: Goshen Biblical Seminary. Distributed, in photocopied form, by Cokesbury, Co-op Bookstore, Duke Divinity School, 1983.

———. *The Christian Witness to the State.* Newtown, KS: Faith and Life Press, 1964, reprinted in 2002 by Herald Press.

———. *For the Nations: Essays Public and Evangelical.* Grand Rapids: Eerdmans, 1997.

———. "Fuller Definition of 'Violence'". John Howard Yoder Collection, Historical Manuscripts, 1–48, Box 02, File 16, Mennonite Church USA Archives. Goshen, Indiana (MCA-G).

———. "How H. Richard Niebuhr Reasoned: A Critique of *Christ and Culture*," in *Authentic Transformation: A New Vision of Christ and Culture.* Eds. Glen H. Stassen, D.M. Yeager, and John Howard Yoder, 31–89. Nashville: Abingdon Press, 1996.

———. *The Original Revolution: Essays on Christian Pacifism.* Scottdale, PA: Herald Press, 1971; reprinting by Wipf and Stock Publishers, Eugene OR, 1998.

———. *The Politics of Jesus: Behold the Man! Our Victorious Lamb.* 1st ed. Grand Rapids, MI: Eerdmans, 1972.

———. *The Politics of Jesus: Behold the Man! Our Victorious Lamb.* 2d ed. Grand Rapids, MI: Eerdmans, 1994.

———. *Preface to Theology: Christology and Theological Method.* Grand Rapids: Brazos Press, 2002.

———. *The Priestly Kingdom: Social Ethics as Gospel.* Notre Dame: Notre Dame University Press, 1984.

———. "Reinhold Niebuhr and Christian Pacifism." *The Mennonite Quarterly Review* 29 (April 1955): 101–17.

———. *The Royal Priesthood: Essays Ecclesiological and Ecumenical.* Ed. Michael G. Cartwright. Grand Rapids, MI: Eerdmans, 1994.

———. "Second Draft of 'Theses' on the Definition of the Free Church Vision." John Howard Yoder Collection, Historical Manuscripts, 1–48, Box 02, File 14, Mennonite Church USA Archives, Goshen, Indiana (MCA-G).

———. *What Would You Do? A Serious Answer to a Standard Question.* Scottsdale, PA: Herald Press, 1992.

"Yoder Suspended." *The Christian Century* 109, no. 24 (August 12, 1992): 737.

Young, James. *Writing and Rewriting the Holocaust: Narrative and the Consequences of Interpretation.* Bloomington: Indiana University Press, 1988.

Index

About the Author

Cynthia Hess holds a Ph.D. in theology from Yale University and has published articles on Anabaptist theology, peacemaking, and religiously motivated terrorism. Currently, she is consulting study director for the Institute for Women's Policy Research in Washington, D.C., where she conducts research on religion, feminism, and public policy.

Breinigsville, PA USA
07 December 2010
250778BV00001B/5/P

9 780739 119457